"*Chicken Soup for the Surviving Soul* will not only comfort and inspire cancer survivors and their loved ones, it will comfort and inspire anyone breathing. It's mandatory reading!"

Wall Amos
"The Cookie Man"

"*Chicken Soup for the Surviving Soul* is a great pick-me-up book. We all go through tough times in our lives. The inspiring stories in this book show us all that we can get through these events and even learn from them—that is the secret of surviving!"

Dan Jansen
Olympic gold-medal speed skater

"Yes! This wonderful book teaches us that one can make cancer a triumph instead of a tragedy! We can find the blessings . . . the lessons to be learned . . . the strength we never knew we had. I know . . . cancer was one of the most empowering 'gifts' in my life."

Susan Jeffers, Ph.D.
author, *Feel the Fear and Do It Anyway* and
End the Struggle and Dance with Life

"Over the past 14 years of providing psychological and emotional support to thousands of cancer patients, we have discovered that there are significant therapeutic benefits from interacting with other cancer patients. *Chicken Soup for the Surviving Soul,* a wonderfully inspirational book, introduces the cancer patient to many others who understand every nuance of the cancer experience."

Harold H. Benjamin, Ph.D.
founder and president, The Wellness Community

D0011866

"These stories will take you by the hand and take you by the heart, and show you how much each of us can do."

W. Mitchell, CPAE
author, *The Man Who Would Not Be Defeated* and
internationally recognized expert on change

"I loved this wonderful, heartwarming book. It reminded me of all the people I have worked with since 1974. Reading it was like sitting in a hundred support groups. You leave feeling you've shared something important, something of yourself."

Elise NeeDell Babcock
founder, Cancer Counseling Inc.
and author, *When Life Becomes Precious*

"*Chicken Soup for the Surviving Soul* shows us what all the blood tests, X rays and MRIs cannot possibly reveal—the true nature of the surviving soul. Through the horror of cancer, these heroes have found the honor of everyday life. By sharing their stories with us, they fill us with the power not only to survive but, indeed, to thrive. Besides cancer patients, their families and health-care givers, anyone who's had so much as a broken nail or a broken heart should read this book."

Robert Wollman, M.D.
Holy Cross Hospital Cancer Center

CHICKEN SOUP
FOR THE
SURVIVING SOUL

101 Stories of Courage and Inspiration from Those Who Have Survived Cancer

Jack Canfield
Mark Victor Hansen
Patty Aubery
Nancy Mitchell, R.N.

Health Communications, Inc.
Deerfield Beach, Florida

We would like to acknowledge the following publishers and individuals for permission to reprint the following material. (We exercised due diligence but were unable to locate the copyright holders for the story on page 2. Please contact us if you are the copyright holder of this item.)

The Soul Menders. Excerpted from her book *Animals as Teachers & Healers: True Stories & Reflections,* by Susan Chernak McElroy. ©1996 New Sage Press.

From on Chemo to on Camera. Reprinted by permission of The Candlelighters Childhood Cancer Foundation. ©1995 by *The Candlelighters Childhood Cancer Foundation Youth Newsletter.* All rights reserved.

You Can Teach an Old Dog New Tricks. Reprinted by permission of Howard J. Fuerst, M.D. ©1996 Howard J. Fuerst, M.D.

The Boy and the Billionaire. Reprinted with permission from the October 1991 *Reader's Digest.* ©1991 by The Reader's Digest Assn., Inc.

Hope. Reprinted by permission of Commune-A-Key Publishing. ©1994 William Buchholz, M.D.

(Continued on page 355)

Library of Congress Cataloging-in-Publication Data

Chicken soup for the surviving soul : 101 stories of courage and inspiration from those who have survived cancer / [compiled by] Jack Canfield . . . [et al.].
     p. cm.
    Includes bibliographical references (p.).
    ISBN 1-55874-402-9 (trade paper). — ISBN 1-55874-403-7 (hardcover)
    1. Consolation. 2. Suffering. 3. Courage—Case studies. 4. Cancer—Patients—Case studies. 5. Terminally ill—Psychology. 6. Terminally ill—Family relationships. I. Canfield, Jack, 1944- .
    BV4910.33.C48   1996
    362.1'96994—dc20   96-13843
                                        CIP

Publisher: Health Communications, Inc.
              3201 S.W. 15th Street
              Deerfield Beach, FL 33442-8190

Cover design by Andrea Perrine Brower

With love we dedicate
Chicken Soup for the Surviving Soul to
Linda Mitchell—a survivor, and Patty and
Nancy's mother—who originally suggested that
we compile it. She spent hundreds of hours
reading over a thousand stories and poems
in the creation of it and gave us the
encouragement to continue when we thought
it would never come to completion.
Chicken Soup for the Surviving Soul
would not exist without you!

We also dedicate it to
Jeff Aubery, Patty's husband, who
spent the last six months of this project as
virtually a single parent with their son J.T.
while Patty worked to complete it.

No Road Too Steep

There is no path
so dark,
nor road so steep,
nor hill so slippery
that other people have
not been there
before me
and survived.
May my dark times
teach me to help
the people I love
on similar journeys.

Maggie Bedrosian

Contents

3. ON ATTITUDE

4. ON FAITH

5. ON LOVE

6. ON SUPPORT

Foreword

I was quite honored when asked to write the foreword to *Chicken Soup for the Surviving Soul*. I have been so touched and inspired by the first two *Chicken Soup* books that my foreword may turn out to be longer than the book. On the other hand, I realized that I could also write a one-word foreword. What is the one word? Love. I could quote all the great spiritual leaders to emphasize this point, but I think you, dear reader, know what I am saying, or you wouldn't be reading this book.

When we see an event that has an emotional impact upon us, one of our choices is to repress the feelings it creates and bury them deep within. In my early years as a physician I was very good at this. I thought I was protecting myself, but I was actually destroying myself. I finally hurt enough to seek healing. Books like *Chicken Soup for the Soul* were part of my healing because when you read, you get in touch with your feelings. You can then express those feelings so that you may heal your life and your body. So read, feel and find healing in these pages.

Learn from the natives—those who have preceded you and found paths to healing. We all have cancer in one form or another—emotional or physical. Ninety percent of the people I speak to say, "Life is unfair." What they are really saying is, "Life is difficult." Yes, but it is difficult for all of us, so therefore, it must be fair. We are all complaining. What this book can reveal to you is not only how to deal with cancer but how to deal with all of life's difficulties and make life a more meaningful experience.

I find as I care for people that they do not lack information about how to live a healthier lifestyle. They lack inspiration that leads to transformation. For some, this inspiration comes when they learn that they have a short time left to live—that they are not immortal. Well, none of us are immortal, and so it is a lot wiser to read *Chicken Soup for the Surviving Soul* and be inspired than to wait until you have a life-threatening illness.

As I have said, my transformation came from my pain as a physician, from storing everything inside me until I suffered from post-traumatic stress disorder, common to so many people in today's society. My patients became my teachers. In helping them learn how to live between office visits, I was also learning about living. So please accept your mortality and find happiness and love. You'll also find that the first person you need to love is yourself.

Who are the best teachers? I find they are the people who don't die when they are supposed to. They will enlighten you about life. They know they are not statistics, nor are they controlled by statistics. A medical student I know got angry when he read that his disease invariably recurs, and seven years later he graduated from medical school with no sign of the "incurable" tumor. Others set out to create a more beautiful world and get so busy they forget to die. They suddenly have permission to quit a job, take off a tie, move to the mountains or seashore, express love, assert themselves, explore a spiritual life, read and do other things they never had time for. They learn the truth of the statement, "Enjoy yourself; it is later than you think." Their enjoyment is not about being selfish. I can't believe how many people think being happy is selfish. I am talking about people who contribute to the world in their own way, not the way someone else decides. As one woman said, "After I had done all the things I wanted to do before I died, I didn't die." Later she wrote, "Now I'm so busy I'm killing myself. Help! Where do I go from here?" I told her to take a nap. She wasn't burning out, she was burning up.

Others decide to leave their troubles to God and then get well. Let the problems in your life be your teachers. Always describe your difficulties with words that express your feelings. Then look at the things in your life that fit the description and heal them. Your life will improve and you will derive physical benefits, too. Remember, life is a labor pain but the pains are not inflicted by someone else. You decide what you go through to give birth to yourself.

We also know that if you experience labor surrounded by caring people, you have far less pain and far fewer complications. So reach out for the help you need. Create a mutual investment society with your family, friends and health care providers. The stories contained here will guide you in how to do that.

These stories will also teach you that life isn't about "Why me?" but "Try me!" You will learn that beating a disease or difficulty isn't only about curing it but about living with adversity in such a way that you inspire those around you. You are a winner because of the way you live, not because you don't die.

Unhealthy guilt, shame and blame have no place in your new life. If you lose your car keys, it isn't because God is punishing you and wants you to walk home, and if you lose your health it also is not because God is punishing you. We (God included) will help you to find your health just as we would help you search for your keys— without guilt or blame.

When you live in the moment, you will be amazed at the change in your life and the inner wisdom you discover. As you will learn from reading this book, transformation is the key. I will let you in on a secret that I only share with readers on how to succeed at transformation.

Your thoughts create chemical changes in your body. What you experience and anticipate alter you. Spend a moment laughing, loving or playing and your body feels different than it does during moments of anxiety, despair or fear.

So what can you do? Behave as if you are the person you want to be. We know from studies that actors and actresses, when simply playing a role, alter their body chemistry depending upon the emotion they are portraying.

When you finish your *Chicken Soup* and are feeling better, decide who you want to be and start becoming your new self. No one can change you but yourself, but a good coach can help bring out the best in you. Let this book be a coach or guide, but seek out other coaches, too.

I will close with one important thought. William Saroyan writes, "Everyone alive is an actor but almost everyone alive is a very pathetic actor." He goes on to say that this is why you are given a lifetime to learn to act like yourself. So forgive yourself when you are not the person you want to be. Then get out your baby picture, look at it and forgive yourself. Then get on with being who you want to be.

One last word of advice—read *Chicken Soup for the Surviving Soul* and become enlightened. And for those of you who do not have cancer but may be a family member, friend or health care provider to someone who does—or just a member of the human species—don't wait until your mortality is threatened to wake up to the lessons of life presented here.

Bernie S. Siegel, M.D.

Acknowledgments

Like the prior volumes of *Chicken Soup for the Soul,* this book took over a year to write, compile and edit. It was a true labor of love for all of us involved, and we would like to thank the following people for their contributions, without which this book could never have been created.

Our families, who gave us the space to do the book and the needed emotional support to persevere through what seemed like a totally overwhelming and never-ending task. You continue to be Chicken Soup for Our Souls day after day after day!

Heather McNamara, who spent countless hours—late into the evening and lots of weekends—reviewing the manuscript and editing each and every draft. Heather, we couldn't have done it without you!

Harold Benjamin, for his insights and brilliance during this project and for taking the time to meet with us to go over the manuscript—giving us much needed feedback.

Dr. Bernie Siegel, for taking time out of his busy schedule to offer advice, insights about the mind-body connection, medical information and much more.

Diana Chapman, for continually sharing her stories, giving feedback on the manuscript and cheering us on throughout the whole project.

Coping Magazine, for allowing us to request stories from their readers in the "letters" section of the magazine.

Joel Goodman, who sent us several pieces on humor that were very helpful.

Anna Kanson at *Guideposts,* for researching and sending us stories. Thank you for your patience! This book would not be complete without you.

Meladee McCarty, who not only read the entire manuscript in record time, but also sent several stories and quotes to help us bring much needed humor to the book.

Michelle Nuzzo, for the encouragement and ideas on where to go for more resources and for editing the initial version of the manuscript. Michelle, you were always there when we needed you!

John Wayne "Jack" Schlatter, who continually sent in wonderfully written stories and supported us throughout the process of this project. You are a true friend, Jack!

Marci Shimoff and Jennifer Hawthorne, coauthors of the forthcoming *Chicken Soup for the Woman's Soul,* for sending in stories from all over the country.

Peter Vegso and Gary Seidler at Health Communications, for believing in us and continually getting our books into the hands of millions of readers. Thank you, Peter and Gary!

Kim Wiele, who kept our general office running during the final phase of this project.

Kimberly Manson Culver, who helped read and grade stories and worked many hours to help complete this project.

Larry Price, who continues to support us and reinforce us with encouragement.

Trudy Klefsted at Office Works, who typed the manuscript in record time and with very few errors. You are a true gem!

Christine Belleris, Matthew Diener and Mark Colucci,

our editors at Health Communications, for their generous efforts in bringing this book to its high state of excellence.

We also want to thank the following people who read the first *very rough* draft of the book, helped us make the final selections and made invaluable comments on how to improve the book: Jeff Aubery, Kelle Apone, Brian Barnwell, Harold Benjamin, Linda Blackman, Diana Chapman, Mona Cohen, Manuel Diotte, Pam Finger, Charles Green, Dr. Robert Grossman, Glenda Hawley, Jennifer Hawthorne, Elizabeth Kapiloff, Kimberly Kirberger, Edd Mabrey, Meladee and Hanoch McCarty, Linda Mitchell, Michelle Nuzzo, Lee Potts, Dr. Ann Raymer, Martin Rutte, John Wayne Schlatter, Marci Shimoff, Bernie Siegel, Janet Switzer, Rebecca Wiederkehr, Dr. Robert Wollman, Monique Djolakian Zgrablich and Kelly Zimmerman.

We also appreciate all the people who sent us stories, poems and quotes for possible inclusion in *Chicken Soup for the Surviving Soul.* While we couldn't use everything you sent in, we were deeply touched by your heartfelt intention to share yourselves and your stories with us and our readers. Love to you!

We are sure in the immensity of this project we have left out the names of some of the people who helped us. For that we are sorry but nonetheless grateful for the many hearts and hands that made this book possible. Thank you all for your vision, your caring, your commitment and your actions.

Introduction

> The stories people tell have a way of taking care of them. . . . Sometimes a person needs a story more than food to stay alive.
>
> Barry Lopez

From our hearts to yours, we are delighted to offer you *Chicken Soup for the Surviving Soul.* This book contains over 100 stories that we know will encourage you to have more hope, empower you to take charge of your life and your healing process, inspire you to give and receive more unconditional love, motivate you to fight and persevere in the face of what may seem to be insurmountable obstacles and odds, invite you to share your feelings, persuade you to reach out for and accept more support, and finally, convince you to live each day more fully and with more humor as you pursue your heartfelt dreams with more conviction. This book will sustain you in times of frustration and challenge, and comfort you in times of pain and suffering. If you let it, *Chicken Soup for the Surviving Soul* will truly be a lifetime companion, offering insight, wisdom and guidance on many areas of your recovery and your life.

During this very challenging time in my life battling cancer, I truly appreciate being able to turn to Chicken Soup for the Soul *for strength and peace.*

Paul

Why This Book?

In January 1995, Nancy and Patty's mother, Linda Mitchell, was diagnosed with breast cancer. Because we have been writing and compiling *Chicken Soup for the Soul* books for the last five years, she suggested that we compile a book with stories from those who have been touched by cancer. At first, the project took off very slowly and we wondered if we would ever complete it. As cancer survivors and their family members began sending us stories of their experiences, and our reading and research on cancer continued, we realized we would finish it and that it would be a great book. But we also realized something else.

When the idea of this book was born, it was about surviving cancer, but as it took shape, we realized that it was really a book about life. In fact, eight million cancer survivors out there have discovered things about life that most of the rest of us have not yet learned. As we continued working on the book, we realized that each story was teaching us what was really important in life. As a result, we deepened our appreciation for the simple things in life—watching the changing hues and colors of the morning sunrise, taking a walk along the beach, listening to music, drinking a glass of fresh squeezed fruit juice, playing with our children and hugging our loved ones. Our families and the love we all share with each other became more and more important to all of us.

At least once a day we sit back and say, "We are so lucky." Because of this book we are not the same people we were. Our priorities are clearer now. We share our feelings more openly, we take our vitamins and herbs more regularly, we eat better, we meditate and do yoga more often, we pray with more conviction and we love with more openness. Our daily disciplines are stronger, our co-dependent behaviors are weaker and our desires to follow our own inner directives are stronger. We laugh more often, take more time for play, worry less about pleasing others and know more clearly than ever that each day is a treasured gift to be lived to the fullest.

> Chicken Soup for the Soul *reawakened me to the fact that life is really too short to hide, it's meant to be lived!*
> Rita Valdez

We thank all of you who have been challenged by cancer because your struggles and insights have deepened our own understandings about life, love and spirituality. We also trust that readers will have the same experience we had as we created this book. We know from sharing the first drafts of this book with many cancer patients, survivors, family members and caregivers that this book will comfort, aid and inspire all who have been confronted with this challenge. It is also our hope that this book will be a wake-up call for those of you who don't have cancer—we hope that it will give you some of the insights without having to personally go through the struggles.

And to those of you who are currently battling cancer, we invite you to let these stories touch you to the depths of your soul and give you the faith, hope and courage to fight and to win because others have come before you and done so. May their stories light your way through the dark nights. We send you our love and our blessings and the love and blessings of all the people who participated in this project. They all care . . . and they know what you are facing and what is possible.

Share These Stories with Others

Sometimes our light goes out but is blown into flame by another human being. Each of us owes deepest thanks to those who have rekindled this light.

Albert Schweitzer

Some of the stories you read will move you to share them with someone else—another patient, survivor, family member, friend or caregiver. When that happens, take the time to call or visit and share the story with that individual. We promise you that you will get something even deeper for yourself from sharing the stories with others.

How to Read This Book

One reader of the first *Chicken Soup for the Soul* book wrote us that she read the book in one sitting of four hours and in that time totally released all the flu symptoms she had! We know that reading this book can affect your immune system. Pretty amazing!

Actually, we don't recommend you read the book all in one sitting. Take your time. Enjoy it. Savor it. Engage each of the stories with your whole being. Reading a book like this is a little like sitting down to eat a meal of all desserts. It may be a little too rich to digest all at once. Take time to experience the story's effect. Listen to the words in your heart as well as your mind. Let each story touch you. Ask yourself, *What does it awaken in me? What does it suggest for my life? What feeling or action does it call forth from my inner being?*

We encourage you to have a personal relationship with every story.

Some stories will speak louder to you than others. Some will have deeper meaning. Some will make you laugh; some will make you cry. Some will give you a warm feeling all over; some may hit you right between the eyes. There is no right reaction; there is only your reaction. Let it happen and let it be.

Write to Us

We would love to hear about your reactions to this book. Please write to us and tell us how these stories affected you. Also, we invite you to become part of this wonderful *Chicken Soup for the Soul* network of upliftment. Please send us any stories and poems you think we should include in future volumes of *Chicken Soup for the Surviving Soul*. See page 338 for our address. We look forward to hearing from you. Until then . . . we hope you will enjoy and be as enlightened by your reading of *Chicken Soup for the Surviving Soul* as we enjoyed and were enlightened by compiling, editing and writing it.

Jack Canfield, Mark Victor Hansen,
Patty Aubery and Nancy Mitchell

1

ON HOPE

Hoping means seeing that the outcome you want is possible, and then working for it.

Bernie S. Siegel, M.D.

What Cancer Cannot Do

Cancer is so limited—

It cannot cripple love
It cannot shatter hope
It cannot corrode faith
It cannot destroy peace
It cannot kill friendship
It cannot suppress memories
It cannot silence courage
It cannot invade the soul
It cannot steal eternal life
It cannot conquer the spirit.

Source Unknown

The Soul Menders

During the first months following my cancer diagnosis, I wouldn't acknowledge any kind of healing but physical healing. I wasn't interested in techniques that could help me cope better or extend my life expectancy by a few months; mere remission or "quality of life" didn't capture my attention either. Full recovery was the only option I would accept, and I was willing to do anything and go anywhere to achieve it.

When my surgeries and radiation treatments were over, I found myself in that frightening twilight zone of life after treatment. The doctors had done all they could and I was on my own to wonder if I'd be alive or dead by the following year. For the sake of my sanity, I tried hard to convince myself and anyone else who would listen that I was doing just fine and that cancer was no death sentence. My motto became, "I don't write off cancer patients." I was ferocious and flailing.

Only two weeks earlier, my lover and I had parted ways. I felt confused and frightened about the future. Alone in bed at night, I looked at the white walls and wondered who would want a 39-year-old cancer patient.

Life in my apartment was dismally quiet. Then, Flora entered my life—a skinny feral kitten about four weeks old, full of ringworms, fleas and ear mites. Shivering and alone under the wheel well of my parked car, Flora looked desperately sick. I grabbed hold of her scraggly tail and tugged. Within seconds my hand was scratched to shreds, but I hung on and brought her hissing and complaining to my apartment. At that point, I realized that my lonely life welcomed the commotion of a tiny, angry kitten who would distract me from my own depressing thoughts.

With the arrival of the kitten, I pulled my energy away from myself and my fretful imaginings and concentrated on healing Flora. Along with ringworms and fleas, she had a terrible viral infection that had ulcerated her tongue, cheeks and throat. I knew all about ulcers in the mouth, so I sympathized wholeheartedly with this miserable condition. It took weeks, but slowly Flora healed, and along the way we bonded. Soon, she was a loving, trusting ball of black-and-white fuzz who met me at my door each evening when I returned from work. The loneliness of my apartment vanished, and I cherished the success of our health venture *together*. Although my own future looked uncertain, success with Flora was something I could achieve.

Only weeks after I'd finally nursed Flora back to some resemblance of healthy kittenhood, she was diagnosed with feline leukemia. Cancer. Her veterinarian gave her the same sorry prognosis my oncologist had given me: Flora would most likely die within a year or two. My response was instant and unconscious. As soon as Flora's vet handed down the diagnosis, I wrote her off as a lost cause. Quickly, my emotional attachment to her ceased as I began protecting myself from the pain of her death, which I knew would come. The veterinarian told me Flora would die and I simply accepted this. I stopped speaking and playing with Flora because when I did, I ended up sobbing hysterically for my kitten. I even found it difficult to look at her. But Flora simply wouldn't let me pull away. When I'd walk past her, she'd chase after me. Her paw touched my cheek hesitantly each night as she curled up next to me in bed, her purr resonant and strong. If my mood was chilly, she seemed not to notice. Flora did what cats do best: she waited and watched.

Her patience finally won out. One night I had an "AHA!" experience about my attitude toward Flora. How could I believe my own cancer wasn't a death sentence when I couldn't see the same hope for her? How could I dismiss any being without dismissing myself? Although I was busy blathering about hope and healing, I knew that I honestly saw myself in the grave.

That realization was a profound turning point for me. While slow in coming, it finally hit me like a downpour of hailstones. How often in my life had I turned away from pain and loss, and from honest feelings? Living at "half-life," I'd put away emotion at the first inkling of loss, and nearly lost myself in the process.

One night shortly after my awakening, I lit a candle for Flora and myself. We sat together looking at the flame, and I vowed to Flora that I would love her with wild abandon for as long as she was with me because loving her felt so good. In loving Flora, I knew I would find a way to love myself as well—poor diagnosis and all. For the both of us, each day of life would be a day we could celebrate together.

I began a quest to heal Flora that included many of the same gems of complementary medicine I attempted on myself. Flora got acupressure, vitamins, homeopathy, music and color therapy, detoxifying baths and unlimited quantities of hugs, love and affection. Her water bowl had tiny, colorful crystals in it. Her collar was a healing green.

Most important in this process, though, was the attitude change I experienced from this "mumbo jumbo," as some of my bewildered friends called it. Healing stopped being so painfully heavy. It became fun, even silly. When I told my friends I might have my house visited by dowsers to seek out and correct "bad energy vibrations," I damn well had to have a highly developed sense of humor!

Over the next few months, I slowly learned that healing is more than heroics over illness. Healing isn't simply an end result; it's a process. Flora helped me reclaim the joy that had died after my cancer treatment and my previous relationship ended. She brought me tremendous peace with her quiet, trusting presence. Finally, as I saw Flora healed, loved and cherished, I knew I honestly held the same hopeful vision for myself.

Flora is sleek, happy and seven years old today. Her last three tests for leukemia have been negative. At the time of my "AHA!" with Flora, I felt that she was an angel sent to teach me that turning away from love accomplishes nothing.

Susan Chernak McElroy

From on Chemo to on Camera

Faith, Hope, Love.
You need all of the above.
If you want to live, then you've got to be positive.
There's a rumor I got a tumor.
I used to be a dancer, but then I got cancer.
I used to have hair all down my back,
but now it's even shorter than Kojak.
But that is all right,
cuz I'm gonna win the fight.

These are some of the lyrics to my "cancer rap song." I wrote it when I found out in March 1989, at age 18, that I had bone cancer. After almost two years of chemotherapy and eight major operations, including an amputation of my left leg above the knee, six tumors later, I am thankful to say I am clean!

I don't wish cancer on anyone, but I don't ever want to forget what I went through. The physical and emotional pain taught me to really love life with a passion. Suffering produces perseverance, character and hope.

I had quite a bit of fun, too, at the hospital while on chemo. Other patients and I (those who were up to it) gathered for little daily parties while having our chemo or hydration. I remember walking around the hospital with no hair, chopsticks stuck up my nose and in my ears, just to get a reaction from unsuspecting people. Nothing felt better to me than making others laugh and forgetting the pain for a while. I feel that God has used my situation and experience to help others.

This passion to entertain also led me to a career. Before cancer, I was a dancer on *Soul Train*. When I was diagnosed, my doctors told me I would never dance again. I fooled them—I still dance, and with a lot of soul. Two years ago, I started taking acting classes. Southern California, where I live, is where most of the entertainment industry is located. I put off going on my first audition because I didn't want to mess up. Would you believe that when I finally went, I not only got the part, but a lead role on a big show? *Northern Exposure!* They were two of the best weeks of my life. I played a character, Kim Greer, who is training for a wheelchair race in Cicely, Alaska, and gets a sprained elbow. Maggie (Janine Turner) introduces me to Ed (Darren Burrows) so he can try to heal me with native shaman ways.

Here's what a day on the set was like. The night before, I studied my lines. I had to get up really early (sometimes at 3 A.M.) to meet the rest of the cast at 4:30 and travel from Seattle to locations. The interior scenes were shot in Redmond, Washington, and the location shots in the little town of Roslyn (population 850). Halfway through makeup I had to go "block" scenes (go through them for the first time with the other actors). Then it was back to finishing my makeup, followed by shooting the scenes. The latter takes a long time because they shoot scenes from different angles, a number of times, and then they have to "process" and "take." The director was really help-ful and funny, and called me "the girl who acts without acting." After finishing in the early afternoon, I stuck around and watched other scenes being shot. It was very educational.

The cast and crew on that show were so special. I even adopted a "grandpa," the man who drove the makeup trailer.

Two weeks after I got back, the same director called me to audition for a small part on *Beverly Hills 90210*. Later I found out they decided to cast me for a big part instead: as a campus activist, opposite Brandon Walsh. I haven't met any of the *90210* actors yet. Most actors, I find, are very different from the characters they play.

Even though I lost a leg to cancer, I am doing more than I ever have. I learned to snow ski on one leg, and now I race and teach other people to ski. Hey, we don't cross our ski tips!

While I have goals in acting and writing, I have learned, after having cancer, not to take things too seriously. Life is temporary. So while I still have it, I'm going to have fun with it!

Kristine Kirsten

You Can Teach an Old Dog New Tricks

The mind, in addition to medicine, has powers to turn the immune systems around. . . .
Jonas Salk

As a graduate of one of the top 10 medical schools, and after four years of residency at a New York teaching hospital, I was well trained in the science of medicine. I was kind and compassionate; most of my patients loved me, as I them. Yet I adhered to my training—if it "ain't" in the medical literature and if it hasn't undergone rigid double-blind crossover studies, it must be quackery. And so it went for 40 years.

Three months before my 69th birthday, my daughter in California sent me a copy of *Quantum Healing* by Deepak Chopra, M.D., which explores the field of mind-body medicine.

For my 69th birthday, even though I felt great, I had a complete medical checkup. I received a definite diagnosis of far advanced prostate cancer. The professor at the medical school again confirmed the diagnosis. He told me there's no cure, but he could slow down the progress of the disease with hormone therapy and I could live 18 to 24 months.

At the time of diagnosis, I went into shock and depression in spite of heroic support from my wife and children. My two daughters in California entered the picture. Immediately, I started reading books and listening to tapes on healing, started a macrobiotic diet, scheduled a course on meditation, had an appointment with a "cancer psychologist" and started visualizing my cancer's destruction. Not one of these modalities was accepted standard medical therapy, and although I performed them with a huge dose of skepticism, I couldn't stand up to my family's forceful persuasion. I was determined to be a good patient and did all of the above regularly and with an attempt at an open mind.

It is now 51 months later. I am well but not the same person. I have made a 180-degree change in my attitude toward the practice of medicine. From a narrow-minded, tunnel-visioned physician, I am now open to all possibilities. I run cancer support groups and espouse diet, meditation, visualization and psychological support. I receive several telephone calls from cancer patients each week who have heard my story and want to know what they can do to help themselves.

Prayer was added about one year ago. Although I had heard about the power of prayer and although my family had me on multiple prayer lines, I was skeptical until I heard Dr. Larry Dossey speak and read his book *Healing Words*. I now watch for numerous articles on prayer and stories on TV. In my own informal way, I speak to God daily.

My days start with 30 minutes of meditation, prayer and visualization. Shopping and cooking are part of my routine. I eliminated all animal products and fats from my diet and increased the amounts of grains, fresh vegetables and other foods consistent with a macrobiotic diet. I still see a macrobiotic counselor twice a year. Listening to tapes by Dr. Bernie Seigel, Dr. Deepak Chopra, Louise Hay and others intimately involved in the mind-body connection are also part of my daily routine. In my reading, I found many "medical miracles" occurring because of "alternative therapies."

Many of my colleagues still look at me as a "nut case" who happened to be lucky and go into remission from my cancer. Why? They don't know. But I do—I had mountains of love and moral support and I chose to change. It saved my life!

Howard J. Fuerst, M.D.

The Boy and the Billionaire

There is no such thing as no chance.

Henry Ford

His sense of humor set Craig Shergold off from the other children. A natural entertainer with an exuberant personality, he loved making people laugh. His greatest joy was putting on wigs and funny hats and staging comedy skits for family and friends at his home in the London suburb of Carshalton.

Craig brought the same buoyant energy to soccer. But in the fall of 1988, his coach noticed a change in the nine-year-old's normally aggressive play. "He seems to have slowed up," the coach told Craig's father, Ernie.

Craig complained of earaches, and his mother, Marion, noticed that his eyes blinked repeatedly when he watched television. He seemed listless, but the family doctor blamed that on Craig's grief over the recent death of a beloved grandmother. As the weeks passed, however, Craig became more and more subdued.

At Christmas, Craig did not even want to ride his new bicycle. This time the doctor blamed Craig's problems on an ear infection. Antibiotics did not help.

A couple weeks later, Craig suffered a bout of vomiting. Marion demanded an immediate hospital appointment, and a specialist put Craig through a series of tests. Then he ordered a brain scan.

Afterward, Marion and Ernie were ushered into a doctor's office. "I'm afraid I have bad news for you," the doctor said. "Craig has a brain tumor." Marion was speechless; Ernie bowed his head.

The tumor, the doctor continued, was lodged in a very dangerous spot: near the top of the brain stem, which controls breathing, heart rate and blood pressure.

An ambulance carried Craig to the Great Ormond Street Hospital in central London, and tumor surgery was soon scheduled. Marion didn't want to tell her son, fearing she'd crush that indomitable spirit. But she had always been truthful with him, and she didn't want to break that trust. She sat at her son's bedside and held his hand. "Craig, do you know what you have?"

"I think so, Mum." He mentioned a character from his favorite TV show who had a brain tumor. "I think I've got what she's got," Craig said.

Marion nodded. "I want you to be very brave," she murmured.

"I will be."

Holding his stuffed elephant for luck, Craig was wheeled toward the operating room on January 17. Marion and Ernie were at his side. Softly, Marion sang "I Just Called to Say I Love You," one of Craig's favorite songs.

Kneeling in the hospital chapel, Marion remembered when she and Ernie first learned that she was pregnant after 10 years of trying. They organized a big celebration at the restaurant where Marion worked as a waitress. Marion led everyone in the singing, dancing and laughing. When Craig was born on June 24, 1979, the joy continued.

Now she pleaded for her son's life. *Lord, Craig's not ready for you. I won't let you take him because it's not his time yet.*

Her prayers seemed unanswered. After hours of surgery, the surgeon reported that he could not remove all of the tumor because of its dangerous location. Two weeks later the dreaded news in the pathology report indicated a malignant teratoma, an aggressive cancer of the brain. After his recovery from surgery, Craig received further treatment, but his death seemed all but inevitable.

Marion quit her job so she could stay with her son in the hospital. Ernie, a truck driver, came after work in the evenings. One or the other was by the boy's bedside 24 hours a day.

Craig received so many get-well cards from family, friends and soccer team members that his doctor joked, "You ought to go for the *Guinness Book of World Records.*"

Shortly before transferring to The Royal Marsden Hospital, where he would undergo chemotherapy and radiation treatments, Craig received a taped get-well message from his favorite TV personality. Hearing this, a national newspaper published an article on this plucky boy fighting for his life. Soon other newspapers, along with radio and television, picked up the story. Craig became "Our Kid Courage" to the British press.

Craig's medical condition worsened, however. His legs and left arm were weaker, his speech slow and deliberate, his vision blurred. For all his pain, though, Craig never lost his sense of humor. He even joked about the baldness caused by the chemotherapy. "Knock, knock," he would say. "Who's there?" a visitor would respond. "Ad-air," Craig answered. "Ad-air who?" "Ad-air once, but now I'm bald!" came the punch line.

The fact that so many people cared gave Craig hope. One night in the hospital, his strength sapped by chemotherapy, Craig fought against the sadness he felt.

"Mum," he said, "I'll think about the cards. Every time I do, it makes me feel better." In September, in an attempt to build Craig's morale, the Shergolds told the press he would try to establish a Guinness record for most cards received.

Days later, a small truck pulled up outside the Shergold home, carrying several large sacks of cards. The outpouring led to more publicity—which generated thousands more cards. He received cards from Margaret Thatcher, Prince Charles, George Bush, Ronald Reagan, Mikhail Gorbachev and two of Craig's idols: Michael Jackson and Sylvester Stallone.

Craig started having real hope of beating the record for most cards collected (1,000,265) held by another English boy. This gave him a sense of purpose, made his condition something more than a cruel twist of fate. In fact, so many cards poured in that Craig received his own "selection box" at the central post office in London, making him the first person in British history designated like a city for mail processing.

On November 17, 1989, the big night arrived. Craig, although shaky, was allowed to go to the local soccer club for the ceremony. As 300 people gathered around, the local post office manager presented Craig with card number 1,000,266—the record breaker. As Craig said thank you, everyone sang "For He's a Jolly Good Fellow."

Some 3,800 miles away, in Charlottesville, Virginia, John Kluge received letters from friends. A soft-spoken man of 77, Kluge is a billionaire who made his fortune in the communications business. Kluge's friends wrote him about Craig and all his get-well cards. They urged Kluge to send a card, too.

As Kluge considered mailing a card, an inexplicable feeling came over him. Amid all the attention focused on the card campaign, he couldn't help wondering: Had every medical possibility been explored? Was there some treatment he could arrange for the boy?

While Kluge had donated millions to worthy causes, he had never given money to an individual. He didn't want to start a precedent. And he didn't want to raise false hopes for Craig's family. Still, he couldn't shake the idea that there might be some hope for Craig.

Kluge phoned a close friend, Dr. Neal Kassell, professor of neurosurgery at the University of Virginia Health Sciences Center. "Neal," he asked, "could you contact the Shergold family? I have the feeling something important might have been overlooked. I'll pay any expenses."

Unable to reach the Shergolds by phone, Kassell air-expressed a letter on August 7. Days passed, and the Shergolds did not answer. His letter, of course, had disappeared into millions of others. Since breaking the record, the number of cards skyrocketed to over 26 million.

Craig was in and out of the hospital regularly. On September 20, Craig's physician, Dr. Diana Tait, asked Marion and Ernie to come to her office. The news was not good. "The latest scans show Craig's tumor is growing again," Tait said. The outlook was bleak. The Shergolds were devastated. This time they avoided telling Craig the news.

The next morning, to get her mind off the situation, Marion decided to open some of Craig's get-well cards. From the stacks of envelopes, Marion plucked the air-express packet containing Kassell's letter. As she read it, her hands trembled. "I can't believe this!" she cried.

Marion called Kassell immediately and told him of the discouraging prognosis. Kassell said he could promise nothing, but added that his medical center had recently purchased a "gamma knife," a new instrument that fired high-energy radiation beams directly into brain tumors. "This might offer a possible treatment for Craig," he said.

"I'll request the scans from Craig's doctor."

When Ernie returned home after work, Marion handed him the letter. "I think God may have given us a miracle," she said.

When he received the brain scans, Neal Kassell leaned toward the light box for a closer look. In the center of Craig's brain, he saw a gray, egg-size tumor that compressed his midbrain area and squeezed the brain stem. Kassell's hopes sank. The tumor was too big to be knocked out by the gamma knife.

Moreover, the mass appeared to branch out and invade surrounding tissue. This seemed to confirm the lab finding that the tumor was malignant. If true, Kassell realized, Craig could never be cured.

Besides, he thought, if he operated, Craig had a one-in-five chance of dying as a result of the surgery. And even if the operation succeeded, he wondered, what would Craig really gain? A few months of life?

Kassell called Kluge with the bad news. "Some things are beyond medical help," he said.

"Are you absolutely sure you can't treat it?" Kluge persisted. "Please think about it some more."

Kassell began searching within himself. The father of three girls, he asked what he would want for them in a similar circumstance. He realized he would give them a fighting chance—despite the risks.

Kassell spoke to the Shergolds in late November. "I might be able to help your son," he said. The surgical risks were great, the benefits chancy. All he could do, Kassell said, was surgically remove as much of the tumor as possible and hit the remainder with the gamma knife. This might buy Craig some time. Kassell suggested the couple ponder their alternatives over Christmas and let him know their decision after the first of the year.

For Marion, the decision was agonizing. She didn't

want to put Craig through any more pain. Ultimately, she and Ernie decided to let Craig make the decision.

"Mum," he said, "no pain, no gain."

Surgery was scheduled for March 1 at the University of Virginia Health Sciences Center. That morning, Marion and Ernie stood at their son's bedside as Craig reassured them. "I'm going to be all right, you'll see."

Moments later, as orderlies wheeled him toward the operating suite, Craig, clutching his stuffed elephant, called out, "I love you, Mum and Dad." He then began singing, "I Just Called to Say I Love You."

Kassell removed a two-inch oval of bone from the top of Craig's skull. Carefully separating his cerebral hemispheres, then splitting the band of fibers joining the two halves, Kassell found the grayish-white tumor almost in the exact center of the brain. It was encapsulated by a membrane—which had not shown up clearly on the scans. *Good,* Kassell thought, *the tumor is much more contained than I had dared hope.*

Kassell sliced open the membrane and began snipping and suctioning out the tumor. Moment by moment, his excitement mounted. This tumor did not appear malignant. Could it have somehow changed character since the British lab analysis two years earlier? The more he cut away, the more convinced he became that Craig might beat the odds.

Three hours into the operation, one of his resident physicians grew concerned that Kassell was moving too deep into Craig's brain. "Don't go in there," the resident cautioned.

Kassell paused for a moment. The operation had been a big gamble from the start. Now, as he looked through the operating microscope and saw the final remains of the mass nestled in Craig's brain, he knew he had to gamble again. He went even deeper.

Kassell left only one small section, mostly scar tissue, in a very risky area. The tissue appeared dead, incapable of ever regrowing.

The surgery took more than five hours. Kassell did not need the gamma knife. Drained and exhilarated, he left the operating room and went to tell Craig's parents the good news. Marion leaped up and kissed him.

In the intensive-care unit, Marion leaned over Craig's bedside and whispered, "Craig, the cancer is gone. All gone."

Craig's eyes flickered open, and he smiled.

Craig's recovery was remarkable. His speech became faster and clearer immediately. He pronounced words that had been impossible for him before the operation. Two days after surgery, when Kassell walked into Craig's room, Craig said, "Doc, you're supercalifragilisticexpialidocious"—and broke out laughing.

Lab tests found no trace of malignant cells in the tumor tissue. No one would ever know for certain what eliminated them. The important thing was that Craig's tumor was benign.

A few weeks later, John Kluge came to the hospital to meet the Shergolds. When the businessman entered the room, Marion grasped his hand and thanked him. "You are our guardian angel," she said.

Kluge handed Craig a two-headed quarter. "This way," he said, grinning, "you'll never lose."

Then Craig presented a gift to Kluge: a mounted photograph of himself in a triumphant "Rocky" pose taken by his mother several months earlier. In it, Craig wore boxing trunks and gloves; an American flag hung in the background. The inscription read: "Thank you for helping me win the biggest fight of all."

John Pekkanen

Hope

As I ate breakfast one morning, I overheard two oncologists conversing. One complained bitterly, "You know, Bob, I just don't understand it. We used the same drugs, the same dosage, the same schedule and the same entry criteria. Yet I got a 22 percent response rate and you got a 74 percent. That's unheard of for metastatic cancer. How do you do it?"

His colleague replied, "We're both using Etoposide, Platinum, Oncovin and Hydroxyurea. You call yours EPOH. I tell my patients I'm giving them HOPE. As dismal as the statistics are, I emphasize that we have a chance."

William M. Buchholz, M.D.

Amy Graham

Where there's life, there's hope.

Marcus Tullius Cicero

After flying all night from Washington, D.C., several years ago, I was tired as I arrived at the Mile High Church in Denver to conduct three services and hold a workshop on prosperity consciousness. As I entered the church, Dr. Fred Vogt asked me, "Do you know about the Make-a-Wish Foundation?"

"Yes," I replied.

"Well, Amy Graham has been diagnosed with terminal leukemia. They gave her three days. Her dying wish was to attend your services."

I was shocked. I felt a combination of elation, awe and doubt. I couldn't believe it. I thought kids who were dying wanted to go see Disneyland, or meet Sylvester Stallone, Mr. "T" or Arnold Schwarzenegger. Surely they wouldn't want to spend their final days listening to Mark Victor Hansen. Why would a kid with only a few days to live want to come hear a motivational speaker? My thoughts were interrupted. . . .

"Here's Amy," Vogt said, as he put her frail hand in mine. There stood a 17-year-old girl wearing a bright red and orange turban to cover her head, which was bald from all the chemotherapy treatments. Her bent body was frail and weak. She said, "My two goals were to graduate from high school and to attend your sermon. My doctors didn't believe I could do either. They didn't think I'd have enough energy. I got discharged into my parents' care. . . . This is my mom and dad."

Tears welled in my eyes; I was choked up. My equilibrium was shaken. I was totally moved. I cleared my throat, smiled and said, "You and your folks are our guests. Thanks for wanting to come." We hugged, dabbed our eyes and separated.

I've attended many healing seminars in the United States, Canada, Malaysia, New Zealand and Australia. I've watched the best healers at work and I've studied, researched, listened, pondered and questioned what worked, how and why.

That Sunday afternoon I held a seminar, which Amy and her parents attended. The audience was packed to overflowing with over a thousand attendees eager to learn, grow and become more fully human.

I humbly asked the audience if they wanted to learn a healing process that might serve them for life. From the stage it appeared that everyone's hand was raised high in the air. They unanimously wanted to learn.

I taught the audience how to vigorously rub their hands together, separate them by two inches and feel the healing energy. Then I paired them off with a partner to feel the healing energy emanating from themselves to another. I said, "If you need a healing, accept one here and now."

The audience was in alignment and we shared an ecstatic feeling. I explained that everyone has healing energy and healing potential. Five percent of us have it so dramatically pouring forth from our hands that we could make it our profession. I said, "This morning I was introduced to Amy Graham, a 17-year-old, whose final wish was to be at this seminar. I want to bring her up here and let you all send healing life-force energy toward her. Perhaps we can help. She did not request it. I am just doing this spontaneously because it feels right."

The audience chanted, "Yes! Yes! Yes! Yes!"

Amy's dad led her up onto the stage. She looked frail from all the chemotherapy, too much bed rest and an absolute lack of exercise. (The doctors hadn't let her walk for the two weeks prior to this seminar.)

The group warmed up their hands and sent her healing energy, after which they gave her a tearful standing ovation.

Two weeks later, she called to say that her doctor had discharged her after a total remission. Two years later she called to say she was married.

I have learned never to underestimate the healing power we all have. It is always there to use for the highest good. We just have to remember and use it.

Mark Victor Hansen

Wild Bill

I always thought I'd live to be 83! Why that age, I don't know, but now I'll be grateful to make it to 58. When I am 58, Rachel will be 12—old enough to understand what is happening. Not that it is ever easy to lose a mom—even when "Mom" is really an aunt.

Actually I am grateful for each day. Every morning when my alarm goes off, I lie in bed a few minutes. Whatever the weather, I am happy to be able to stretch my legs out, give my dog a pat, and thank God for another day. My favorite days are those when the sun streams in through my lace curtains, but I even like the sound of rain pattering on my window or the wind moving the trees against the side of the house. It is in the morning that I feel the best. It is morning that gives me hope.

Nearly two-and-a-half years ago, a tumor on my left adrenal gland ruptured in the middle of the night, leaving me near death from excessive blood loss. As I lay on the operating table, I thought of my three grown children, of my unfinished business, but mostly I thought of Rachel, whom I'd left crying hysterically in the living room of our home when the paramedics hauled me off. Somehow,

I made it through the surgery, made a rather astounding recovery and returned to work in six weeks. Rachel and I resumed our lives.

The tumor was strange. No one could clearly say what it was except that it was malignant. Five major medical centers couldn't identify it. I began calling it "Wild Bill."

For a little more than two years, I did well except for a bowel obstruction that responded to non-surgical treatment. Every three months I visited an oncologist in Chicago who did tests that I passed with flying colors. After a while, I did not think much about "Wild Bill."

After New Year's this year, I began feeling excessively tired, my back ached more than usual, and I was running a low-grade fever. I was admitted to the hospital for tests. Everything from active TB (I had been exposed at work) to an arthritic condition was considered. As part of the work-up, an MRI of my abdomen was ordered. The test was supposed to take 45 minutes to an hour but stretched into two hours and beyond. My mind and heart raced and tears flowed into my ears like a river. It was the first time I cried over my illness. I could not wipe my tears away and no one could hold my hand, but I knew what the MRI showed was not good. The next day a needle biopsy of part of the tumor confirmed that "Wild Bill" had returned. I felt lost and depressed. All I could think about was Rachel.

A rather smug but well-qualified surgeon came to see me. "We'll do an exploratory lap and see what's what and remove what we can, but I give you no guarantees," he said.

When I woke up from the surgery, I listened to those five disappointing hopeless words: "We couldn't get it all." They've yet to explain exactly what they could and could not get. Depending on whom I talked with, I had at least four different versions. Maddening.

At first my recovery was fraught with a terrible sadness that I couldn't shake. I got thinner and thinner and I couldn't eat. I couldn't sleep either and hurt too much to toss and turn, so I would lie like a board all night. Even though my family, friends and coworkers all rallied around me, I could not feel any hope. I even wished I had died the night the original tumor ruptured.

I can't say I snapped out of it. It was more like a gradual slide. I started chemotherapy and even though I was fearful of that, it gave me hope. Reading books was very positive for me—I read of countless hopeless cases who recovered or lived way beyond expectations. Lived good lives, too. I began feeling better. With the help of a friend and a kind priest, I learned how to pray again. Now Rachel and I pray together every night. I stopped wishing I had died that terrible night in December of 1992.

Over the last couple of years, so many good things have happened that I would have missed. My older son published his first book, my younger son's acting career took off again and my daughter and her boyfriend built a beautiful home for their future together. Rachel learned to ride her bike and to read. I resumed an old friendship with a cherished friend. Things that I took for granted were important to me. My sister moved back from California and we can see each other so much more often. If I had died that night I would not have been here to say goodbye to my own dad, who died last fall. Rachel may have never recovered from the trauma and suddenness of it all.

What I really know now is that we never really know. So now when I wake up, I am grateful for whatever time I have. I feed the birds and stray cats. I pick flowers and plant some. I call my sisters and friends. I help Rachel with her homework. I feel stronger each day. "Hope" is the word, I guess; that is so important now. If I have hope, I can do my best to do all I need to do to get well.

Mary L. Rapp

Kids with Cansur

*Children have a remarkable talent for not tak-
ing the adult world with the kind of respect we
are so confident it ought to be given. To the irri-
tation of authority figures of all sorts, children
expend considerable energy in "clowning
around." They refuse to appreciate the gravity
of our monumental concerns, while we forget
that if we were to become more like children our
concerns might not be so monumental.*

Conrad Hyers

The setting remains vividly etched in my memory: My
husband, Craig, and I are sitting in a brightly sunlit consultation room at the Mayo Clinic. A children's cancer
specialist opposite us delivers as compassionately as possible the devastating news that our six-year-old son has a
particularly deadly form of advanced cancer. Craig and I
look at each other in shock, then I ask tearfully, "Is Jason
going to die?" The doctor offers a somber reply.

Years have passed, yet I can still hear those words, the
doctor's grave tone, his hesitation before answering, "If I

am to be honest, I have to tell you . . . probably yes."

I suppose it's natural for parents to avoid thinking the unthinkable. Who imagines that their home will be invaded and their child abducted by this vicious intruder? Certainly I didn't. Children's cancer, I thought, happens only to those wonderful, strong women canonized in the *Ladies' Home Journal*. At the time of Jason's diagnosis, I had never known anyone, adult or child, with cancer. I was a housewife and mother of four, one an infant daughter; Craig, a hardworking husband and father. We were a typical, close-knit family from rural Worthington, Minnesota. Our son's sickness crashed into our lives like a flaming meteor through the roof of our cozy home. To say we felt unprepared and overwhelmed is an understatement.

Our son didn't die. Two grueling years of intensive chemotherapy, radiation and surgery—not to mention our flooding heaven with prayers—saved his life. Today, Jason is a healthy, active teenager, a loyal Dan Marino and Larry Bird fan who rattles the walls of our home with rock music. He is also the author of *My Book for Kids with Cansur*. (The title's misspelling was as close as he could come at the time.) Jason wrote it toward the end of his medical treatment, when he seemed well on the way to recovery.

I remember the two of us curled up on a sofa one afternoon, flipping through a children's book about cancer, written by a young patient. As in several others we'd read together on the subject, at story's end the little boy died. "What a terrible book!" Jason fumed. "Why do they always write books and make movies and stuff about kids who die? Didn't they ever hear about somebody like me, who had cancer and grew up and lived? Why don't they write a book about that?"

Stuck for an answer, I suggested, "Maybe you ought to write your own book, Jason," never dreaming that he actually would.

"Well," he said with a huff, "maybe I ought to."

Several months later, I was washing dishes when Jason bounded into the kitchen. "Here it is," he said as he casually handed me his "book," scrawled in a yellow spiral notebook. I admit, I'd expected some cutesy, silly little thing; nothing too profound. But as I turned the pages, tears streamed down my face. "If you get cansur, don't be scared," my son advised, "cause lots of people get over having cansur and grow up without dying." I found it remarkable that a child could possess such insight about a disease many adults struggle to understand.

That night I gave it to my husband to read. Closing the cover, Craig wondered aloud, "Wouldn't it be something if we could get this into the hands of other mothers and fathers who are just starting down the path we're finishing up?" If our son's surviving cancer had taught us any lesson, it was that nothing is impossible.

You'd be amazed at your resiliency when your child's welfare is at stake. I love it when people say to me now, "Gee, Geralyn, you're such a strong person. I could never survive something like that." Of course they could. As parents, you do whatever you have to for your ailing child. You don't have a choice! Our family's story is by no means one of heroism, just of human beings' remarkable ability to adapt and survive.

If there was one mistake my husband and I made, it was not realizing how a child's cancer impacts every family member, and that each has his or her own capacity to cope. Relatives, friends, teachers and co-workers all feel the profound effects of a youngster's catastrophic illness.

Cancer researchers have made enormous and rapid progress, especially in the field of childhood cancers. Had Jason been stricken 20 years earlier, he almost certainly would have died within a matter of weeks. In the mid-1960s, only one in five kids survived cancer, as opposed to one in three by the mid-1980s. Like most parents of children with cancer two decades before, we would have been gently advised to prepare for our son's imminent death. Today's cure rate has reached an all-time high of more than two in three, with recent medical advances further supporting hopes for a child's recovery.

It takes love and faith to emerge from such an experience intact, and it's not easy. I must tell you that when this happened to Jason and our family, I thought our lives would always center around his disease and could never, ever be pieced back together again. But as time passed, that proved not to be the case. Our lives have evolved and we realized we were not alone. People do withstand this crisis. There can be life after children's cancer. We are proof of that.

Geralyn Gaes

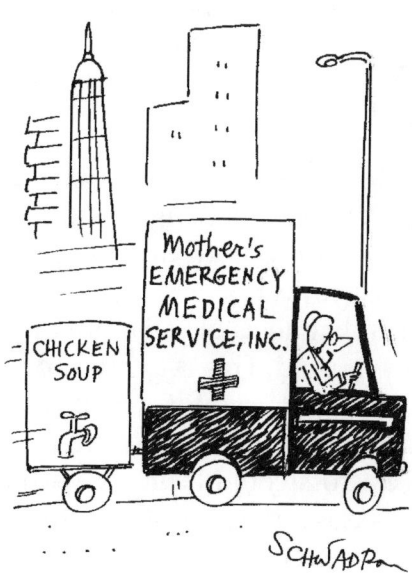

Reprinted with permission from Harley Schwadron.

Cancer Has Been a Blessing

You gain strength, courage, and confidence by each experience in which you really stop to look fear in the face. You are able to say to yourself, "I have lived through this horror. I can take the next thing that comes along."

Eleanor Roosevelt

"I want you to know right now, don't try to save my breast and put my life in danger, I can live without a breast." I said those words to my oncologist when diagnosed with breast cancer.

I received this diagnosis of inflammatory breast cancer when I was 38 years old. This is a rare and very aggressive type of breast cancer. It accounts for only 1 to 6 percent of all breast cancers and it has a very high rate of recurrence. I was told the doctors could treat me with chemotherapy and put me in remission for probably three to five years. Most likely after the remission, I would have a recurrence, and at this time they know of nothing that can eradicate the cancer. I told the oncologist I wanted the best treatment for my disease that he knew of. I was willing to do anything. Three to five years' remission was *not* acceptable to me. My doctor told me of this aggressive protocol that was being used at the Dana Farber Cancer Institute in Boston that he would recommend for this type of breast cancer.

The protocol required that I have strong chemotherapy for three days a week, every other week for four cycles. Then I would be admitted to Dana Farber for very high doses of chemotherapy and a bone marrow transplant. I would then need to have a modified radical mastectomy followed by six weeks of radiation. Needless to say, I was in shock. I knew this was going to be bad, but I never expected it to be this bad. When he said I needed a bone marrow transplant, I knew my cancer was more serious than I had thought.

After I was diagnosed by the surgeon and before I consulted with an oncologist, I took my then five-month-old granddaughter for many walks in her carriage. We walked and I talked to her. When I was outside with her, I could think more clearly, and I made many decisions while with her. She may have only been a baby, but she was a great listener and I decided then that I could not keep on crying, asking God, "Why me? Why now?" It would have been very easy to feel sorry for myself, but I realized all those thoughts were not productive. I realized that I had to face this head on and fight for the chance to be a part of my granddaughter's life for many years to come. I told her that I was not going to go anywhere and that her "Grammy" was going to be here for her. She is one of the major reasons that I was prepared to fight and willing to do all that I could to beat this cancer. When the doctor asked me if I would be willing to go through this very difficult protocol, I didn't hesitate to say yes.

After a consultation at the Dana Farber Cancer Institute in Boston and acceptance into its protocol, I began chemotherapy in July of 1993. In November, I entered Dana Farber for the high-dose chemotherapy and a bone marrow transplant. Fortunately, I didn't have too many serious side effects from the transplant and I came home on Thanksgiving. I had set a goal for myself to be home with my family for my favorite holiday of the year. After recovery, I had a modified radical mastectomy early in January of 1994. At that time the pathology on my breast and lymph nodes came back with *no residual cancer cells.* This was the best news we could have hoped for. I then had six weeks of radiation. In April, I finished the protocol and in June went back to work after being on sick leave for a year.

Cancer has changed me in many ways. My whole outlook on life is so much clearer now. I didn't realize how much I took health and life for granted until I thought mine was in jeopardy. Now every day is a gift and I am grateful that I have this time. When you have had cancer, your future is so uncertain. I faced the fact that I might die before I reach old age; therefore, I need to make the most of the time I have now. I appreciate my life so much more now that I have had cancer.

I also realize how strong I am, even though I never thought of myself that way. So many people tell me how strong and courageous I have been through all this and now, as I look back on it, I realize I did what I had to do to survive, as would most people. I didn't think of it as courage that made me do what I had to do, I thought of it as survival. But now that I can look back and reflect, I realize that it did take strength and courage to face cancer the way in which I did—courage and strength that I didn't know I had.

One of the most important aspects of my life that helped me conquer breast cancer is a loving and supportive family. Without them, I am not sure what my outcome would have been. I had so much to live for and was not ready to leave them yet, and I was not ready for them to go through life without me. I wanted to be a part of their lives for many years to come. Knowing that they were all there for me, supporting me, helped me to get through all the treatments and all the hard times when I wanted to give up. They were my source of strength and support, my motivation and inspiration.

One day, if any of them are faced with the same diagnosis, they will do the same. I hope that I set an example for them and that I have inspired them. I also hope that they gained knowledge and strength from my experience. I strive to help other people who have to go through this same procedure, to give them information and educate them about this treatment. It helps to know that someone else may benefit from my experience. My mother taught me that everything happens for a reason. She feels that I was given cancer so that I could help someone else. Today, that is my mission, to help others get through this and to look at me and think, *If she got through breast cancer and survived, then I can, too.*

Cancer is such a dreaded disease and it has robbed us all of so many wonderful people. I have lost a grandfather, two aunts and a cousin—all to cancer. Even though it was terrible to lose them, it also gave me strength. I saw what they all went through and it made me stronger. I was determined not to go through what they had gone through.

The day before I went to Dana Farber for the high-dose chemotherapy and the bone marrow transplant, I went to the cemetery to visit my cousin, who was just four years older than I when she died just a few weeks earlier. I knelt at her grave and vowed to her that I would go to Dana Farber and get through this transplant for her as well as for me. I know that if she could have gone through what I was about to, she would have done it willingly if it meant she would live. When she died, people worried about me, but I told them all that I was going to gain strength from her death because she was an inspiration to me when I was diagnosed.

While I would never want to go through a cancer diagnosis again, it does not seem so frightening to me now. I have learned that you can battle cancer and win. Although cancer is terrible, for me it has also been a blessing. I am stronger and better now. I have so much self-confidence and faith in myself now. I now know that I can do anything. I can face anything that is thrown at me. I just have to face it head on and take it one day at a time.

It has been almost 18 months since I had my last radiation treatment and I feel great. Greater now than I have in a few years. At times I feel so great, I am almost euphoric, like I am walking on air. It is wonderful to be healthy again. When I was diagnosed, I felt like most people who are diagnosed with cancer. I felt like I had just been handed a death sentence. Cancer meant death, but now I know differently. You can survive breast cancer.

Kimberly A. Stoliker

Cancer and Career Choices

Discovering the ways in which you are exceptional, the particular path you are meant to follow, is your business on this earth, whether you are afflicted or not. It's just that the search takes on a special urgency when you realize that you are mortal.

Bernie S. Siegel, M.D.

At the tender age of 27, I had been married for six years, enjoyed a flourishing career in the food service industry, was about to buy my first home and was the delighted daddy of two beautiful and remarkable children—a boy and a girl.

At age 43, I was two years divorced, owned a prosperous small business, was in the process of purchasing a new domicile, had found love again and was on the verge of remarriage, thus becoming the proud papa of two more adorable children.

Fifteen years later, the children are all grown up and still wonderful, but all else is gone—marriages, homes, businesses. However, I am now a successful real estate salesman, secure in the knowledge that given time I will recoup all.

Now let me sort out my list of things to do: continue making loads of money, find Ms. Right, buy a new home, raise a new family and I'm complete, right? Not! I will always believe that at this point, in my thinking, God threw up his hands. "Enough already! What do I have to do? Strike my child with lightning? Wait, I've got it—a life-threatening illness will point him in the correct direction. Either that or it will kill him. What to do, what to use? Cancer, that's it, cancer. But what kind? Not just life-threatening, also a threat to his manhood; he'll heed that. That's it, prostate cancer. I am all-knowing."

I can come up with no other answer than that Divine Providence generated my urge to get a complete physical, and my additional need for reassurance that I wasn't losing my manliness—okay, okay, potency—led me to discover I had a diseased prostate. Further tests indicated the cancerous condition was operable, but if I did not take decisive action and allowed the cancer to spread, I would be counting the months I had to live and those days would be filled with more hospital stays plus painful, debilitating treatments. My doctors explained all the options—at least the ones medical science had to offer— but the best one seemed to be complete removal of the offending organ. I would not be the natural father to any more children, since it is the prostate gland that produces semen, which carries the sperm. I could live with that— literally. Additionally, any of the curative options could possibly render me incontinent, even impotent. Just what I needed to hear, but I could live with that, too.

At this point, I must mention that we all have several special gifts or talents—there is also usually one outstanding one. I had already acknowledged and expressed my entrepreneurial, social and family skills. I'd been there, done that—but my most special gift, the uninhibited expression of my fertile imagination through creative writing and film mediums, was completely neglected. I sensed God's impatience, so as they wheeled me into the operating theater, I made a pact with my Maker. I would do my part to completely actualize the blessings of my God-given gifts, talents and abilities if He would just allow me to come out of this alive. I vowed I would no longer waste time doing over again what I had already shown I could do well; I would no longer resist the pursuit and development of my artistic talents since, obviously, that is what I was put here to share.

In keeping with my deal, I'm writing this brief account to tell you the cancer had not spread, the operation successfully removed the disease from my body, and my most recent tests show I am still cancer-free. The threat of that terminal illness has compelled me to do what I would not do before—create to the best of my ability, driving me toward the completion of my first novel and onward to a film of my own written work.

At the moment, I have a regular job that I refer to as "my day job." It keeps food on the table, a roof over my head and even affords me a few luxuries, such as the best equipment to help produce my chosen work and the time to do the same. I have never been happier. The thrill and the ecstasy that fill my life come from knowing that I am honoring my true essence and seizing this second chance to fulfill my life's destiny—triumphantly expressing, in writing, my uninhibited passion. Matter of fact, that's exactly what I'm doing right now.

Robert H. Doss

It Is the Best of Times

On April 10, 1995, my 36-year-old brother, Jonathan, heretofore in good health, had a seizure while eating lunch at work. Fortuitously, the office manager heard a thump, went to my brother's office, and found him collapsed on the floor. She immediately called 911. I babysat my two young nieces, Heather and Elizabeth, as my mother and Jonathan's wife, Cindy, rushed to the hospital. We were told that he was conscious, and that tests would be performed to determine the cause of the seizure.

The first phone call confirmed that the usual tests had turned up negative, but that there was a gray area on the brain scan that they wanted to double-check. "Brain tumor," I thought, as I watched his two young children play. When Cindy called again, she confirmed the unthinkable.

I told Heather that her daddy had to stay in the hospital overnight. She started to cry. I assured her that he would be okay. What else could I say? He had to be okay. He would be okay.

We packed up the girls and hurried them over to our house for the night. Brain tumor? It was hard to comprehend. Sitting in our kitchen, eating noodle soup, the oldest began crying again. I picked her up and she clung to me, her tears subsiding somewhat. The youngest, still at that age of sunny self-centeredness, didn't comprehend the enormity of the situation. Later, we ate popcorn and watched *The Lion King*. The oldest said she would feel better if I slept in the same room with her that night.

One day the week before his collapse, Jonathan had awakened feeling somewhat sick, disoriented and sore. He and Cindy attributed the symptoms to dehydration, and the back pain to carrying his oldest child on his shoulders at the zoo. "Brain tumor" is not something that comes to mind. How could he have known that he had a seizure in his sleep the night before? Within a few days, he had felt better.

The information we had on his condition so far was positive for a brain tumor. It was huge. The size of a large egg or a small orange, they said. The size and shape of it indicated that it was benign, non-cancerous. It must have been, as it grew inside my scientist brother's brain for an estimated two to three years with no significant symptoms.

Surgery was scheduled for Thursday, with a surgeon held in high esteem. I visited my brother on Wednesday to bring presents and flowers and wishes for his recovery from myself and our sister, who was living in another state. He looked awful and seemed disoriented. He said that the tumor was attached to a membrane adjacent to the brain. At least it wasn't attached to the brain itself, I thought.

On Thursday, our mom and dad, Cindy and I went to the hospital early to wish Jonathan well before he was prepared for surgery. It would take between two and five hours, they said. Two hours if the tumor was soft and could be more easily removed. Five hours if the tumor was hard and had to be removed more carefully and slowly. Once the surgeon began the operation, he discovered the tumor was hard and attached to the brain. A four-inch-by-four-inch portion of the skull had to be removed. The operation took the full five hours.

Afterward, within the hour, we were able to see him. Jonathan looked amazingly well for someone who just had brain surgery. Although his head was swathed in bandages, not even all his hair was removed.

By Saturday, he was ready to leave the hospital. On Easter Sunday, I went to his house for dinner. The house looked like a florist's from all the flowers that had been sent. At least 20 guests were in attendance. Cindy planned a wonderful dinner, giving him a break from the cooking, which he usually does. Heather and Elizabeth returned from spending time with their other grandparents and were obviously happy to have their daddy home again. I made a joke that he was a rarity—a rocket scientist who had brain surgery.

As a person on the far side of "Generation X" (born in 1963), sometimes I get tired of hearing about the "good old days" when so many things are better now. These are the best days there are, and my brother is living proof of that.

Joanne P. Freeman

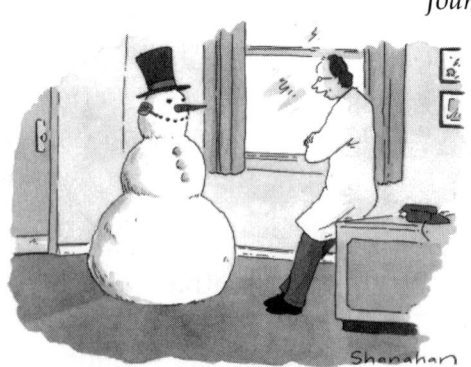

"Good news—those lumps were just coal."

Drawing by Shanahan; ©1996 The New Yorker Magazine, Inc.

READER/CUSTOMER CARE SURVEY

If you are enjoying this book, please help us serve you better and meet your changing needs by taking a few minutes to complete this survey. Please fold it & drop it in the mail.
As a thank you, we will send you a gift.

Name: _____

Address: _____

_____

Tel. # _____

(1) Gender: 1) ____ Female 2) ____ Male

(2) Age: 1)____ 18-25 4)____ 46-55
2)____ 26-35 5)____ 56-65
3)____ 36-45 6)____ 65+

(3) Marital status:

1)____ Married 3)____ Single 5)____ Widowed
2)____ Divorced 4)____ Partner

(4) Is this book: 1)____ Purchased for self?
2)____ Purchased for others?
3)____ Received as gift?

(5) How did you find out about this book?

1)____ Catalog 2)____ Store Display
Newspaper
3)____ Best Seller List
4)____ Article/Book Review
5)____ Advertisement
Magazine
6)____ Feature Article
7)____ Book Review
8)____ Advertisement
9)____ Word of Mouth
A)____ T.V./Talk Show (Specify) _____
B)____ Radio/Talk Show (Specify) _____
C)____ Professional Referral _____
D)____ Other (Specify) _____

(6) What subject areas do you enjoy reading most? (Rank in order of enjoyment)

1)____ Women's Issues/ 5)____ New Age/
Relationships Altern. Healing
2)____ Business Self Help 6)____ Aging
3)____ Soul/Spirituality/ 7)____ Parenting
Inspiration 8)____ Diet/Nutrition/
4)____ Recovery Exercise/Health

(14) What do you look for when choosing a personal growth book?
(Rank in order of importance)

1)____ Subject 3)____ Author
2)____ Title 4)____ Price
Cover Design 5)____ In Store Location

(19) When do you buy books?
(Rank in order of importance)

1)____ Christmas
2)____ Valentine's Day
3)____ Birthday
4)____ Mother's Day
5)____ Other (Specify _____

(23) Where do you buy your books?
(Rank in order of frequency of purchases)

1)____ Bookstore 6)____ Gift Store
2)____ Price Club 7)____ Book Club
3)____ Department Store 8)____ Mail Order
4)____ Supermarket/ 9)____ T.V. Shopping
Drug Store A)____ Airport
5)____ Health Food Store

Which book are you currently reading? _____

Additional comments you would like to make to help us serve you better.

_____

_____

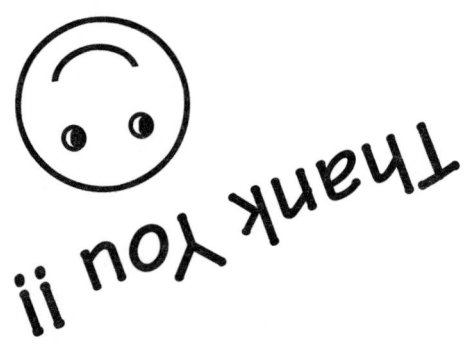

Thank You !!

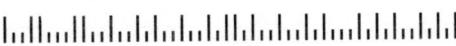

2

ON COURAGE AND DETERMINATION

If I were asked to give what I consider the single most useful bit of advice for all humanity it would be this: Expect trouble as an inevitable part of life and when it comes, hold your head high, look it squarely in the eye and say, "I will be bigger than you. You cannot defeat me."

Ann Landers

Up the Down Slope

Come to the edge.
No, we will fall.

Come to the edge.
No, we will fall.

They came to the edge.
He pushed them, and they flew.

Guillaume Appolinaire

If you could see me now—a confident 18-year-old cruising the University of Colorado campus in Boulder—you'd never believe I'm the same withdrawn, quiet girl I was five years ago. Back then, I was about as shy as a teenager could be. Maybe because I wore thick glasses and was self-conscious, or because my parents had recently divorced—who knows? It got so bad that when I tried out for the track team, I quit before tryouts were over, just so no one would laugh at me. Instead, I'd come home after classes and make a beeline for the TV. I knew the reruns of *Gilligan's Island* like the back of my hand.

But then, during the spring of my eighth-grade year, my left knee started to ache. I thought I'd twisted it or something, so I didn't pay much attention to it. But the pain got worse. At a friend's slumber party I was so uncomfortable I ended up sitting in a reclining chair all night. So my father took me to our family pediatrician, who took an X ray and then called my dad into his office.

I was in the other room, but I heard the doctor talking through the wall. "We don't know yet," he said. "It could be an athletic injury. . . or some sort of tumor."

My Aunt Roselle had once had a tumor, but an operation had fixed that. So I figured I'd just have some quick surgery and then I'd be fine, too.

The day my mother and I went to the hospital for more X rays, Mom's best friend, Peggy Hanson, came along with us. She's known me since I was a baby and she's sort of like an aunt to me. A nurse put the X ray results on a screen. "See here?" she asked, pointing to a white area on the leg. "That's what's making your knee hurt."

Soon a man came in and introduced himself as Dr. Chang. He poked around my knee a little, then looked at my chart. Finally he spoke, slowly and gently.

"Adrienne," he said, "Your leg's been hurting because you have a tumor. If this tumor were to spread to the rest of your body, it could be very dangerous; you could even die. Fortunately I think we've caught it in time to keep it from spreading. But you'll probably have to undergo chemotherapy, and we may have to amputate your leg. I'll know better after we do some more tests."

My mom sucked in her breath and started to cry. Peggy, though, stayed cool and composed, and so did I. I still kept hearing the words *maybe* and *possibly*, which, to me, meant "probably not." And I didn't realize then what an amputation actually involved.

After a minute or two Dr. Chang left us, and that's

when Peggy stepped in for my mom, who was still crying. "Adrienne," she said, "could you handle an amputation?"

"Sure," I said, "I don't see why not."

"You have a family and a lot of friends who love you," Peggy said. "But most of all, you have the good Lord. We'll all be right here to help you through this." Peggy was strong. I admired her strength and drew from it.

The next day I went for a bone scan, and the day after that, an arteriogram (they injected dye into my artery to see where the tumor was). I had to lie flat for 24 hours, and when I finally was allowed to get up, I had to go into the operating room for a biopsy. That was not the best day of my life.

The doctors decided that an amputation was necessary. First, though, I'd have a month of chemotherapy. Little by little, with each visit to the hospital I learned more about that tumor. I found out that most people don't die from my disease since amputation and chemotherapy usually take care of it, and that if you're in remission for five years, you're probably free of it forever. I also found out that only three people in a million get it.

Meanwhile, I was missing a lot of school, and one night my friend Janice called me. "Everybody's talking about you," she said. "Some of the kids say you're bald and you're having both legs amputated. Someone even said you had only a few weeks to *live*."

Janice had no idea how upsetting her phone call was. I was the *shy* one, the girl who hated when people looked at her or talked about her. I remembered how Peggy said I was lucky to have friends and God to help me through this; well, my friends had "helped" by making me into the latest gossip. As for God's role, I was thoroughly confused. I had just started chemotherapy, which made me tired and sick, and in less than a month my leg would be amputated. Was I being punished for something?

Then one night something happened that completely changed the way I looked at the whole thing—and changed everything else about my life as well. It was around 2:00 A.M., and I was lying on the living room couch. I slept there because there was less space to move around in and agitate my leg. The room was dark and quiet, and I was all alone.

I was thinking again about how only three people in a million get this type of bone cancer, three in a million. And it ran through my mind that there were more than three quarters of a million people living in the Denver metropolitan area. That meant that only about five of them would ever have what I had. The thought sort of stunned me. All of a sudden those figures made me feel, well— special. *Suppose God isn't punishing me at all?* I said to myself. *Suppose he has deliberately chosen me?* Let me tell you, that theory got my mind racing. I wasn't sure why I might have been chosen or how it might be a good thing, but I started looking at the cancer in my leg differently. I knew I could deal with it. When I woke up the next day, I felt a new sense of courage. I was ready to face it.

That courage led me to do things I never would have done before—me, the gal who had been afraid to try out for the track team. A few days before my operation, I called my guidance counselor. "Ms. Larson," I said, "would it be possible for me to get together with a group of students during sixth period tomorrow?"

The next day I sat in a classroom and watched it fill up as more than 40 kids filed in. "I asked you all to come here because I want to tell you exactly what's wrong with me," I told them. "In two days, my left leg will be amputated six inches above the knee. After that, I'll have more chemotherapy. My hair will fall out, and I'll be very sick for a while, but I will come back to school in the fall. If you have any questions, you can ask. It doesn't bother me."

At first it was so quiet I could hear myself breathe. Finally, one girl spoke up. "Will you have an artificial leg?"

"Yes," I answered.

"Will you have your real foot?" piped someone else.

I laughed, and one by one the rest of them laughed, too, as they realized the absurdity of the question.

"Well, I sort of doubt it," I said. "I'll just have a bar or something. You probably won't want to see it."

"Aww, come on, Adrienne," said another girl. "We don't care what you look like. We just want you back."

Well, that made me feel great, and by now everyone was much more at ease. And somehow I wasn't at all nervous about speaking anymore.

Time flew after that, and before I knew it, the Thursday of my surgery arrived. By 7:00 A.M. I had a crowd around my bed: June, my youth-group minister from Littleton United Methodist Church; "T," the hospital social worker; and of course, Mom and Peggy. (My dad came later, when things were calmer.) Then T pulled out a little package and handed it to me. "This is from Janelle's mom," she said.

Janelle was a friend of mine who'd also had bone cancer. I tore open the wrapping paper. Inside sat a little brown teddy bear, and across his chest was a message. It read, "Teddy bears are a symbol of love and friendship, and I hope this one reminds you that there are a lot of people who care about you and are hoping that everything will turn out okay for you." I thought back to Peggy's first statement about my having friends to help me through this. Peggy was right—and right about my family and the Lord, too.

I was shaking with nervousness as they wheeled me down to surgery, but when I woke up in the recovery room afterward, I was strangely calm. In fact, I felt a huge sense of relief. The worst of it was over; now I could start doing things again. In a sense, I could start my life over.

As soon as I felt well enough to get out of bed, I began talking to other kids in the hospital. I was surprised to find how bored I was by my usual TV shows. Now I made an effort to meet people and make friends. Oddly enough, it came easily now; everyone seemed curious about my condition, and just answering their questions gave me something to talk about. I felt my former shyness slipping away like an old piece of clothing that no longer fit. When Children's Hospital asked me to be in their telethon, I happily accepted.

I'd been in my church's youth group since I was little, and as soon as I felt well enough, I began going back. We met every Sunday night, and sometimes we'd play volley-ball or other games. When I first came back, the kids seemed uncomfortable; they didn't want me to feel left out. But I didn't mind; I'd stand on the side and cheer them on.

Once I started feeling stronger, though, I wanted to play, too. I knew I couldn't put pressure on my artificial leg, but I developed a fine sense of balance on one leg. One night, before I could reconsider, I took off my pros-thesis. "I'm coming in," I called. The kids stopped the vol-leyball game and stared at me, but when I got the leg off and hopped out onto the court, they all smiled and cheered. Later that summer, when I went to a special camp for cancer patients called Sky High Hope, I did everything from rock climbing to horseback riding. Soon every new sport became a challenge. Especially skiing.

Rick Rakestraw, an instructor from Children's Hospital, showed me how I could ski by using one ski and two out-riggers—poles with little skis at the ends. The second I went down that first bunny hill, I knew this was the sport for me. I wasn't afraid at all.

Before long, I joined the school flag squad, I learned to ride a bicycle and I went out for the swim team. I thought back to track team in eighth grade, how I'd quit before I'd even given it a fair try. So now, even though I was slow and it was tough, I stuck with it. By the end of the season, I was winning races.

But through it all, skiing remained my first love, and one day I was lucky enough to meet Paul DiBello, a skier on the U.S. Disabled Ski Team. Before I knew it I was training with Winter Park's own handicapped competition program, which is coached by Paul. It's been the ultimate challenge; every minute is a thrill. Next year I go out for the national team. Watch out! I'm coming!

Sometimes when I'm drifting in a ski lift over a snow-covered mountain, I think about how if I hadn't had cancer, I probably wouldn't even be skiing—or swimming, or biking, or anything.

Getting sick was no joy, and I certainly wouldn't want to go through it again, ever. But I did have family and friends and God to help me see that something good can come out of just about anything. Cancer gave me a courage I'd never had before—the courage to conquer with one leg what I once couldn't even face with two.

Adrienne Rivera

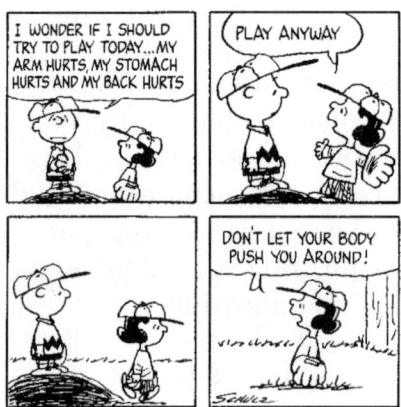

Peanuts ©1996. United Feature Syndicate.
Reprinted by permission.

"Never Give Up!"

Sir Winston Churchill took three years getting through eighth grade because he had trouble learning English. It seems ironic that years later Oxford University asked him to address its commencement exercises. He arrived with his usual props. A cigar, a cane and a top hat accompanied Churchill wherever he went. As Churchill approached the podium, the crowd rose in appreciative applause. With unmatched dignity, he settled the crowd and stood confident before his admirers. Removing the cigar and carefully placing the top hat on the podium, Churchill gazed at his waiting audience. Authority rang in Churchill's voice as he shouted, "Never give up!" Several seconds passed before he rose to his toes and repeated: "Never give up!" His words thundered in their ears. There was a deafening silence as Churchill reached for his hat and cigar, steadied himself with his cane and left the platform. His commencement address was finished.

Speaker's Sourcebook II

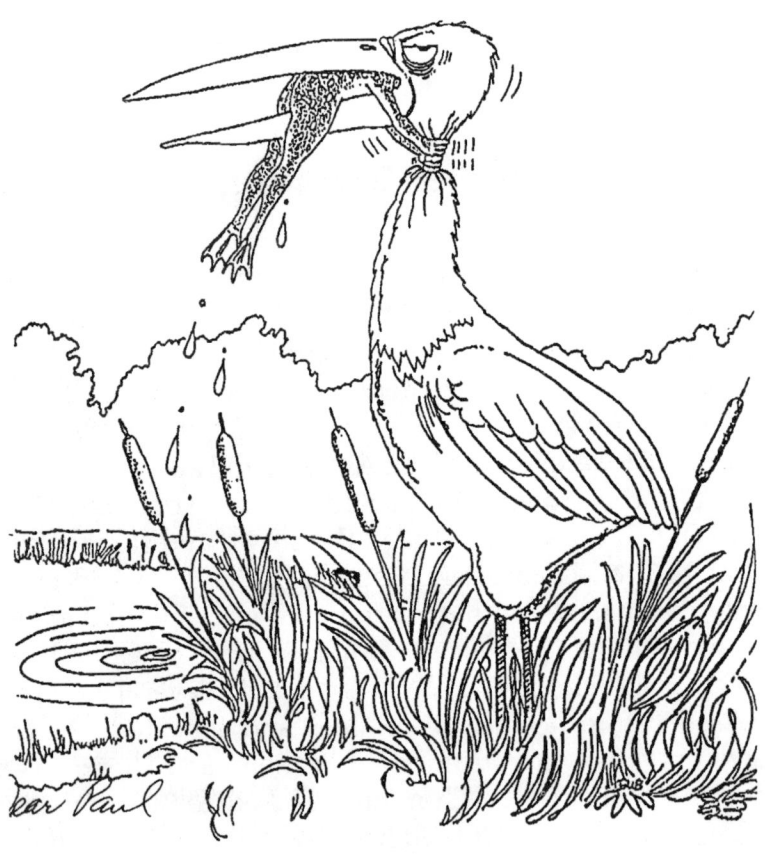

Don't EVER give up!

Not Without a Fight

Life is what happens when you're busy making other plans.

John Lennon

My life until July of 1992 was unusually full. The mother of seven children, I also held a full-time teaching position and was a re-habber of aging houses. I was positive, I was invincible and depended heavily on my Irish luck to remain so. It occurred to me in early spring that I had not had a mammogram in several years. Some weeks later, my eldest daughter received word from Loyola University in Chicago that she was the recipient of a fellowship to pursue her master's degree. She invited me to accompany her to Chicago to find an apartment. I was excited because with my family size, we seldom have the opportunity to spend long periods of time alone together. Checking my calendar, I realized that I had an appointment at 10 o'clock the same day for my checkup. I was tempted to cancel and reschedule. However, I thought I'd just run in, do my thing and then I'd leave for Chicago right away.

Everything proceeded normally until the technician returned to the room and said, "Mrs. Brindell, I'd like to take another picture of your left side." Irritated to have to endure another uncomfortable procedure, I hesitantly agreed. Time was passing quickly, and I found myself watching the clock. Didn't these people know that I had made an important date with my daughter? I didn't want to disappoint her. I considered dressing and walking out. After all, it wasn't my fault if the technician couldn't get a clear picture! For some reason, I remained there and again the technician returned saying, "The doctor wants another picture."

This time he wanted it deeper. "Good grief," I told her, "if this machine is the latest in technological inventions from Sweden, don't they have any full-busted women there? This is really beginning to hurt!" We repeated the procedure five more times. My torso ached and finally I said, "Come on, what's going on here? I've really got someplace to be at one o'clock!"

Suddenly, the kind technician who had been so pleasant until then said very seriously, "Wait right here. I will call in the radiologist." The room became an empty void and time stopped.

The radiologist opened the door slightly to say, "Remember that little lump you had on your left side? Well, it has changed in size and density."

"What does that mean, Doctor?"

"It means that it could be cancer. I'd like to do a biopsy. We'll call you on Monday to schedule." Stunned, I dressed slowly. Not me! No way, not at 48. Life was really just beginning for me. All the really good things were just starting to happen. As I drove home that day, I resolved not to let the morning's events interfere with my Chicago weekend with my daughter. But try as I might over the next few days to forget, I felt that I had a new companion and I was not sure if it was welcome company.

Upon my return to St. Louis, the pace quickened. The biopsy indicated cancer. My husband of 24 years is a devoted man, but when it comes to being emotionally supportive in times of stress, leave him out. The kids, too, continued doing their own thing. I soon realized that if I were going to get through this "mess," I would have to call upon all the inner strength for which we Irish women are so famous. And call upon it I did!

On July 8, 1992, the day of my 25th wedding anniversary, I was wheeled into surgery. I remember saying to my husband, "Well, Bob, some people get to go on cruises on their 25th anniversary, I get to have surgery!" The surgeon came into the room the following day to tell me there were two types of cancer cells present; one was an estrogen-based cell and the other was a very aggressive cell. I knew then I had met my match, but I refused to go down without a fight!

My recuperation was very painful. I couldn't sleep. The pain was incessant. Nor was I able to move my arm. Slowly, very slowly, I began taking charge. I located a physical therapist who gave me exercises to work the arm muscles, I met with a nutritionist to discuss a better diet, and I prepared myself for the radiation therapy that was soon to come.

Crazy as it may sound, the day after I came home, I went to the backyard and began to put in a new sidewalk. Each day, with one arm, I filled buckets with pieces of concrete. I had to test myself. I set goals for myself and worked to achieve them. After all, I had a teaching position to return to in a few weeks and wasn't going to let cancer stop me.

I took radiation therapy every afternoon following a full day of teaching. I tried hard not to miss any work during that time period. I didn't want my colleagues to think that because I had cancer, I was no longer a quality teacher. By October of 1992, I felt I had won the battle!

Then, early December found me back at the surgeon's office for a checkup. We were chatting when he leaned over, touched my neck and said, "How long have you had this lump?" I said, "Oh, about a year. My regular doctor thinks it's an arthritic nodule." I noticed his frown as he suggested that it be removed. My family insisted that I take a day off and follow up on the doctor's suggestion. Another biopsy, what a waste of time! Christmas was right around the corner and I was busy preparing for the holidays.

Once again, I was wheeled into surgery. This time, the diagnosis was thyroid cancer. More stitches, more therapy, more pain. I was down, but not out!

I recall in the solitude of my living room thinking that the first cancer was a fluke, but the second time around told me to get my "house" in order. Then I changed my mind. I decided that it was important to grieve, but if I wallowed in self-pity, any life left to me would be dull.

I set goals again. What did I really want to do with the rest of my life? I have always thought that teaching on the college level would be fascinating. Tomorrow evening, I begin teaching my first class. I feel good about that achievement.

I took positive steps to enjoy the little things. I take the time from doing housework now to go to the kids' soccer games. I like to feel the autumn breeze while my son plays ball. I take joy in the spring as the trees turn green. Simple pleasures bring great happiness. This summer, while waiting for a baseball game to begin, I walked down to the nearby creek, took off my shoes and walked in the water. As the cool, clear water passed over my feet, I realized how simple God's plan is, yet how complicated we humans make his earth.

I have learned compassion. I now know that in the spectrum of time, all humans are working toward an ultimate goal. I have an inner sense of peace that was not there before. Nothing really matters but those truths that exist in one's own heart. You need only look deeply to find them.

I try hard not to be sad. When difficulties arise, I am confident that they last for a brief period, then things get better.

Would I have learned this lesson without cancer? Probably not! What lies ahead for this survivor? Life, learning and love.

Mary Helen Brindell

Nintendo Master

When I first saw you, I thought—Nintendo Master. There was this intensity about you. Your piercing blue eyes and the way your hands moved rapidly along the control buttons were subtle hints of your expert skill.

You didn't appear too different from all of the other video-crazed 10-year-olds out there, but you were. I guess the fact that it was summer, and we were both stuck in the oncology ward of the hospital cruelly betrayed the normalcy with which you tried to present yourself. Or maybe it was the fact that we were prematurely robbed of the innocence of childhood, and it comforted me to know that there was someone else out there just like me. I can only speculate, but all I know for sure is that I was drawn to your energy and zest for life.

That was the summer of my first post-cancer surgeries. The doctors were trying to fix my left hip joint, which had shattered under the intense bombardments of chemo-therapy treatments. It wasn't the only thing that had shattered. I had misplaced my usual optimistic attitude about life and was surprised at how nasty I could be. This did not help me endear myself to anyone.

My surgery went "well," the doctors said, but I was in excruciating pain. (The ever-present differing perspective of doctor and patient is an amazing thing.)

I saw you again in physical therapy, realizing only then the extent of what cancer did to you. I wanted to scream, "Let him go back upstairs and play his video games, you idiots!" But I just sat there in stunned silence. I watched you get up and start walking with the aid of the parallel bars. Prior to your entrance into the room, I sat in my wheelchair wallowing in self-pity. I thought, "Wasn't the cancer enough? Now my hip is screwed up, and I really don't care anymore. If I get up, it is going to kill me."

You will never know me, but you are my hero, Nintendo Master. With such courage and poise, you got up on your one remaining leg. Some might have the audacity to call you disabled or even crippled, but you are more complete than many can ever wish to be. After you had your walk for the day, a walk that was perfectly executed on your part, and you were safely tucked into your bed enjoying your video games once again, I decided that it was about time that I got up and took a walk myself. You see, Nintendo Master, it dawned on me then that you had innately known what it takes most of a lifetime to grasp—life is like a game, you can't win them all and yet the game goes on, forcing all to play it. Nintendo Master, you play it better than most!

Katie Gill

Fighting Back—One Man's Battle with a Brain Tumor

When you get to the end of your rope, tie a knot and hang on. And swing!

Leo Buscaglia

He held the drill in his left hand, moved the bit into position, flipped the switch and began working. One hole. Two holes. Then a third. He could have been building shelves or remodeling the basement. But this was no ordinary handyman. He was a brain surgeon, and the holes he was drilling were in my head.

I lay awake on the operating room table, prepped and draped, waiting and listening while the drill bit passed through my skull. There was no pain, only slight discomfort and an audible "pop" each time the drill penetrated the dura (the tough membrane that covers the brain).

The surgeon finished drilling, then inserted a catheter containing five radioactive seeds into each hole. Once the powerful seeds were planted, an X ray was taken to verify that they were in place. When satisfied with their positions, the surgeon stitched up the wounds in my head.

His "project" was finished. My malignant brain tumor was officially under attack.

This nightmare had begun about four months earlier. I was 40 years old and working hard at the time, putting in long hours as a surgical chaplain at Methodist Medical Center in Peoria, Illinois. As a surgical chaplain, I ministered to patients and families before, during and after surgery. During the procedure we moved between the operating room and the waiting room, giving the family information about the status of the operation. This was an excellent way to reduce anxiety and make the surgical experience as positive as possible for loved ones.

Although my job was tremendously rewarding, it also was extremely demanding. My colleagues and I were "on call" 24 hours a day, seven days a week, and during some surgeries, particularly open heart, we could be in and out of operating rooms for 20 hours or more at a time. Working under these conditions, it was not surprising that I had more than my share of headaches. Most of the time I ignored the pain, chasing it away with a couple of aspirins.

But in the spring of 1987, aspirins were no longer doing the trick. And now my vision was slightly blurred, I was misspelling words, and I found myself bumping into things from time to time. Clearly, the stress of my job was getting to me. I decided to see my family doctor for a checkup.

On April 21, I had a routine exam and a battery of blood tests. Neither revealed any problems. On May 7, I underwent an MRI, which revealed the source of my headaches and other symptoms. There was a dark shadow about the size of a golf ball on the left side of my brain.

My family doctor delivered the news as directly and gently as he could. He drew a quick sketch of the brain and indicated where the tumor was located. "You'll have to have a biopsy next week," he explained, "so we know what we're dealing with. In the meantime, I want you to get this prescription filled and take this medicine to avoid seizures." Too stunned to talk or ask questions, I left his office and returned to my own. There I shared the news with my secretary, then drove home—dazed, numb, virtually paralyzed with shock.

Earlier that day my wife, Pat, and our children had gone to visit relatives living in another city. I knew I had to be with them, but was too emotionally devastated to drive myself. The chairman of the pastoral care department and his wife were kind enough to take me. We arrived at my in-laws' home late that night, and as Pat met us at the door, she knew the news was not good.

I can hardly recall what happened next. Monday came; it was time to meet the surgeon. During our brief meeting, he spoke frankly. "The tumor appears to be an advanced form of cancer." He encouraged me to ask questions, but at the time, I had none. I was still too numb to think clearly.

My biopsy was scheduled for the next day, so I was admitted to the hospital that afternoon. Because I'd worked there for seven years, many staff members were friends and provided extra support and attention.

I remember one orderly who took me for a routine chest X ray the evening before the biopsy. We talked as we traveled to the medical imaging department and when we returned to my room, he asked to pray with me. This simple act of love moved me to tears.

After a restless night, I awoke early and prayed, "Dear Lord, please give me the courage and strength to face whatever this day might bring."

It was a grueling day, and the pain only got worse when my surgeon informed Pat and me that I did indeed have a grade III astrocytoma, which meant my cancer was quite advanced, my condition extremely serious. He sat quietly and waited for my response.

A voice came out of nowhere to break the silence. "How long?" it whispered.

"Six to nine months," replied the surgeon. "Maybe a year."

Another long pause . . . then the voice again. . . . "How will it happen?"

"You'll go to sleep one day," he said, "and never wake up."

I closed my eyes and let his words sink in. My death was on the horizon . . . and there was nothing I could do about it.

The surgeon left me alone with Pat, my parents, my sister and brother-in-law. Few words were spoken as we all tried to grasp what we'd just been told.

Following my discharge from the hospital, Pat and I decided to go away together as a couple, to start facing the present and planning for the future. We spent a weekend in seclusion, talking, crying, praying, trying to make sense of it all.

We held each other and talked about our lives together, our children, our shattered dreams. "What will we do?" Pat cried in anguish. "How will we go on? I'm so afraid!"

As I saw my own despair mirrored in Pat's eyes, I suddenly realized that I had to draw on God's strength and love to get through this nightmare. It was as if God said to me, "You are an ordained minister; it is your job to comfort people. Call on My strength now, for Pat and for you, as you would for patients and their families."

I took a deep breath and declared, "I'm going to fight back, Pat. I'm going to have radiation and chemotherapy. I know the doctor has given me no hope for survival, but I can't just let this thing beat me. I want to go on working as long as possible. Working as a chaplain is my ministry, my life! I can feel that God wants me to do this, that he has a purpose for me."

When we returned from our getaway, closer to one another and closer to God, we tried stepping back into a somewhat normal life. We held regular family meetings to keep the lines of communication open. I encouraged everyone—even my seven-year-old son—to ask questions, speak honestly and vent their emotions. At the time, we believed I had virtually no options for cure, but I fought to prolong my life with aggressive chemotherapy and radiation treatments.

During radiation, I used guided imagery techniques to help overcome my fears and anxieties. I imagined a game going on inside my head, and every time the Pac-Man gobbled up another dot, one more piece of my tumor was destroyed.

Just as I was about to wrap up the treatments, my surgeon contacted me about a new procedure being done in San Francisco. He called it "interstitial brachytherapy," and said it involved implanting highly radioactive seeds directly into the brain tumor. I immediately went to the medical center's library and read articles in medical journals, learning all I could about this new hope.

Pat and I discussed this new option with the surgeon, and although it sounded frightening, we agreed I had little to lose by pursuing it. I knew I had to continue striking back at the insidious foe within me. My records were sent to California to determine whether or not I was eligible for the procedure. Then we sat back and waited, afraid to hope, yet unable to give up.

It was more than three months before we received word that I was accepted into the program. We rejoiced at the news.

On September 12, Pat and I flew to San Francisco. We were accompanied by my department chairman, who came along to provide moral support. My surgeon, who hoped to learn the new technique, went on another flight.

The surgery on September 15 went smoothly. The radium seeds were placed in catheters and inserted into my tumor. After a few quick stitches, I returned to my room, where I waited in radiation isolation while my tumor was under siege.

The radioactive attack continued for five days. Then the seeds were removed, and we returned home. As we pulled into the driveway on September 23, I cried at the sight of a cardboard sign hanging above the front door. "Welcome home Dad!" it said in a host of Crayola colors. My children were so precious to me. I had so much to live for.

Back in Peoria once more, I was again challenged to resume a normal life. I rested and recuperated, then went back to work as a chaplain. I had a new perspective on the trauma of surgery and the terror of terminal illness, which made me a more effective chaplain. I also had an important new responsibility—counseling patients and families in the neurosurgery unit, especially those with brain tumors.

My health improved, although I still had headaches, so I arranged to have a follow-up exam.

I received devastating news. I'd have to undergo yet another surgery to remove the now encapsulated tumor and associated destroyed tissue.

I prayed for strength: "Dear God, I have endured much, and I face yet another battle. Please give me the strength to do what I must that I may live to continue your work."

On March 24, 1988, I underwent craniotomy surgery. I was in the hospital for a week.

There were many days when I believed I couldn't hang on any longer. But deep inside I knew I had to hang on, and God, my family, friends and co-workers carried me through. Now, nearly eight years after my initial diagnosis, I'm still here, a living testimony to the powers of faith and medicine.

My peripheral vision is gone. My speech has been affected. I can't always put my thoughts together like I used to.

But I am alive. Despite all my limitations, I've been given a miraculous gift—eight more years of life with my wife and children, eight more years to serve the Lord in my role as a chaplain. I pray that I have many more.

Since my last surgery, I've spent many hours talking to people with brain tumors and training health-care professionals who deal with them. Based on my experiences as both a patient and a caregiver, I believe there are several keys to coping with this devastating illness.

The first is an attitude . . . a desire to fight back. It's difficult to choose to fight, but patients who go on the offensive from day one have a much greater chance of survival than those who retreat in fear.

But fighting back means taking control, and that may seem virtually impossible to some. The only way to gain power over this deadly force is to be smarter than it is . . . and that requires information. I encourage every patient I see to become an expert on his or her illness. Read and ask questions. Join a support group. Immerse yourself in information. Exhaust every possibility in your search for knowledge. The more you know about the challenges you face, the greater chance you have to surmount them.

Although it's critical that patients take charge of their illnesses, it's equally important that they ask for—and accept—help from those around them. There's no glory in going down this path alone. And there's incredible strength to be gained by accepting support from family, friends, clergy, doctors, nurses, social workers and, perhaps most important, others who have had similar experiences. Their help literally can save your life.

My last piece of advice is to "take things one day at a time." When I was in the depths of despair and others shared that time-worn cliché with me, I had to suppress the urge to react with violence. It made me so angry to hear them mouthing that phrase. But the fact is, in order to survive, I had to stay focused on the day at hand. It was far too frightening—and dangerous—to fast-forward to the future. I'll admit there were times when I thought about dying, and the truth is, I still do today. But I firmly believe you must live in the present to secure your future.

As I reflect on my experiences over the past six years, I'm struck by how many positive memories I actually have. Despite the power drills and popping sounds, the skull screws and seizures, my most vivid memories are of the people—many of whom were complete strangers— who loved and prayed and cared for me and my family during our darkest hours. To them and to the world-class team of health-care professionals who fought on the front lines of this battle, I express my deepest gratitude. I am truly blessed, and I thank God for the opportunity to share my blessings with others.

I still minister to patients with brain tumors and their families. As I walk into each patient's room I introduce myself by saying, "Hello! I'm Chaplain Craig. I think we have something in common. . . ."

Reverend Robert Craig

Dare to Dream

Life! What a precious gift from God. What a blessing to be alive in a wonderful, vibrant world of unlimited possibilities. Then, adversity strikes, and this "gift" feels more like a curse. "Why? Why me?" we ask. Yet we never get an answer, or do we? After contracting Hodgkin's disease at age seven and being given six months to live, I triumphed over the odds. Call it luck, hope, faith or courage, there are thousands of survivors! Winners like us know the answer—"Why not us? We can handle it!" I'm not dying of cancer. I'm living with cancer. God doesn't make junk, regardless of what comes our way, and I don't have to be afraid anymore.

In my sophomore year of high school, the class was scheduled to run the mile. I will always remember that day because due to the swelling and scars from surgery on my leg, for two solid years I had not worn shorts. I was afraid of the teasing. So, for two years I lived in fear. Yet that day, it didn't matter. I was ready—shorts, heart and mind. I no sooner got to the starting line before I heard the loud whispers. "Gross!" "How fat!" "How ugly!" I blocked it out.

Then the coach yelled, "Ready. Set. Go!" I jetted out of there like an airplane, faster than anyone for the first 20 feet. I didn't know much about pacing then, but it was okay because I was determined to finish first. As we came around the first of four laps, there were students all over the track. By the end of the second lap, many of the students had already quit. They had given up and were on the ground gasping for air. As I started the third lap, only a few of my classmates were left on the track, and I began limping. By the time I hit the fourth lap, I was alone. Then it hit me. I realized that nobody had given up. Instead, everyone had already finished. As I ran that last lap, I cried. I realized that every boy and girl in my class had beat me, and 12 minutes, 42 seconds after starting, I crossed the finish line. I fell to the ground and shed oceans. I was so embarrassed.

Suddenly my coach ran up to me and picked me up, yelling, "You did it. Manuel! Manuel, you finished, son. You finished!" He looked me straight in the eye, waving a piece of paper in his hand. It was my goal for the day, which I had forgotten. I had given it to him before class. He read it aloud to everyone. It simply said, "I, Manuel Diotte, will finish the mile run tomorrow, come what may. No pain or frustration will stop me. For I am more than capable of finishing, and with God as my strength, I will finish." Signed, Manuel Diotte—with a little smiling face inside the D, as I always sign my name. My heart lifted. My tears went away, and I had a smile on my face as if I had eaten a banana sideways. My classmates applauded and gave me my first standing ovation. It was then I realized winning isn't always finishing first. Sometimes winning is just finishing.

Manuel Diotte

Fulfilling My Dreams

I believe that good is manifested from every experience that comes into our lives. I also believe that there is a purpose for everything, whether we know what it is or not.

A little over a year ago I was diagnosed with breast cancer. At the moment of this disclosure I was devastated. I did my crying for about 24 hours, and then chose to take as much control of my new situation as I could.

This was a disease that happened to other women, but not to me. I see now how ignorant I was. Since that time I have become more knowledgeable about breast cancer, and I am much more aware. I have a new appreciation for life, a common occurrence when cancer strikes.

Maybe it was my wake-up call to smell the roses. Maybe it was what I needed to become more motivated, to go after goals and to accomplish long-thought dreams.

Since I was a child I wanted to be a published author. A desire burned deep inside me to write and to see my words in print. It was my fantasy, one I suppressed because I lacked self-confidence.

As I went through my mastectomy, chemotherapy treatment and later reconstruction surgery, I wrote almost daily letters to my best friend of over 30 years. She is on the other side of the country and writing has been our main means of communication. We often joke that our letters were our therapy as life brought us new and sometimes difficult challenges. My diagnosis was my toughest challenge to date, and she was there with me every step of the way, giving me constant love and support.

Just before I was diagnosed I purchased a home computer. Naturally I used it to write my letters to her. A couple months into the breast cancer experience, I realized that my letters to Rita could be a book. As a self-imposed therapy, while undergoing chemo, I compiled my letters.

Seven months from my diagnosis of breast cancer, my half-completed manuscript was sold. I have since completed it and I am thrilled to say that my first book, *Courage and Cancer, A Breast Cancer Diary: A Journey from Cancer to Cure* will be published in October 1996.

Yet, there still remained some self-doubt in me regarding my ability to write. I had put together a book of prose almost 16 years ago when I was agoraphobic. It was for my eyes only and I had never dared to let anyone else read it. To prove to myself whether the breast cancer book was a fluke or not, I sent a copy of the prose book to my new publisher. I was amazed when the publisher sent me a contract for that one, too. *Love, Fear and Other Things That Cry Out in the Night* will be published in 1997.

I was on a roll and I had no intention of stopping. In less than a year I have sold three books for publication. I have two more manuscripts out for review. And, of course, I have started yet another one.

My breast cancer diagnosis gave me a new life. I would never have consciously asked for this disease, but I am grateful that it has helped me to fulfill my dreams.

Marilyn R. Moody

Chris—One Special Fifth-Grader!

It was Christmas again. The same magic that fills the air every year at Christmastime was in the hearts of most of the fifth-graders on that cold December afternoon—one of the last afternoons before Christmas break. As was the usual custom, the fourth- and fifth-graders were watching a Christmas movie. The magic that was in the air for most was not there for one fifth-grader, who was dealing with a burden much heavier than any 10-year-old should have to deal with.

As the carolers sang, Chris' heart became heavier and heavier by the moment. He sprang from his seat and ran outside and into his mother's car. His mother was a teacher, along with me, at the small rural school. Other teachers encouraged me to go and talk to him. How do you talk to a 10-year-old who knows that he has cancer, that he will probably have to have his leg amputated and face months of chemotherapy treatments? I'm sure he had a nagging worry that he might die.

I was not just Chris' teacher. I shared in the pain and anguish he was going through. It was just last December that magic was certainly not in the air for me, either. That

December I had surgery and was given the news that cancer had been found. Mine had been operable, but I had spent the past year going through three surgeries, two of those within a month's time, and the other six months later. I also had chemotherapy treatments.

How could I talk to him? This was the question in my mind as I slowly, hesitantly, left the building and went out to talk with Chris. About the only thing I could do was hold his hand and cry with him. He asked me questions and I tried to answer in words that he could understand. When I told him that I had to go every three months for checkups, he said that he sure wished that he was to the point of going for checkups. I tried to explain that the things we go through make us stronger people, and that perhaps he would be able to help someone else someday. Finally, we went back into the building that day, two hearts heavy with burdens shared.

In January the dreaded painful day came. The leg was amputated. Chris returned to school a few weeks later. He was soon fitted with a prosthesis. The children at school were fascinated that Chris could take off his leg. They were very understanding and helpful. In addition to coats and hats, it was not unusual to have a leg in our closet. Other students were always ready and willing to bring him his crutches or his leg. Whatever he needed, they were there and ready. It was a tough year, but rewarding to see the caring and giving of the other students.

As winter faded into spring, the chemotherapy treatments took their toll on Chris. He lost all of his hair. For a while, he tried to wear a nice looking wig that his mother bought for him. One very hot, humid day when no air was moving, right in the middle of class, off came that hot wig. It didn't matter what he looked like, at that moment his comfort was more important than his pride. After another very hot day of physical education outside that spring, as he struggled with those crutches, I suggested that he come to the front of the line and get a drink of water. The other students encouraged him to do the same, but he informed us that he would just take his turn like everyone else. The only special privilege he really enjoyed was being able to wear a hat inside the school building to hide his hairless head.

One day an older man who had been a teacher and a principal before retiring came to visit the students and to tell them about a special contest that a civic club was sponsoring. This special man always quizzed the students and talked to them about the importance of patriotism and school. On this particular day, Chris sat there with his hat on. This very patriotic man walked over to him, removed his hat and said, "Boy, take that hat off when you're inside!" As he removed the hat from Chris' head, a look of surprise, sympathy and remorse all filled his face at the same time. Chris just looked up at him, smiled, reached for the hat and placed it back on his head. At that moment I think I felt even more empathy for the man who removed the hat than I did for Chris.

During all the health problems that Chris faced, he never lost his courage or his faith. He and his family began this ordeal having just partially recuperated from a terrible accident five years earlier, in which his father and his grandmother were killed, and Chris was seriously injured. How much must one young man face? I am sure this is a question asked by many people.

Chris and I are both doing fine now. In December, it will be eight years since I had cancer. I feel that I am better qualified as a teacher because of what happened to me. It has helped me to understand and help students who may have family members suffering from cancer or other serious illnesses. I hope I will not have any more students who have to go through anything like Chris had to deal with, but if I do, I'll do my best to help them through it.

In October, it will be seven years since Chris was diagnosed with cancer. We are survivors! Both of us know it was the Lord who brought us through the tough times. Chris will graduate from high school this coming year. He is a very handsome young man who will soon enter college and pursue his career. I am sure he will choose a career that will involve helping others. He is that kind of young man.

Louise Biggs

My Hero

It is Thursday. I hate Thursday. Today, multitudes of parents and children make long trips in order to arrive at this destination . . . hell. It is a crowded and noisy place. It is a place where people do not smile, a place where pain and fear lurk around every corner. I exit the elevator on the fourth floor, turn the far-too-familiar corner, and sit in an uncomfortable chair. People are all around me, yet I am alone. Although my journey has just begun for today, it is not an unfamiliar one. I have been here many times before. Twenty-one grooves in each tile. I have counted them often. I settle myself in my chair because I know it may be some time before my name is called. Suddenly, I hear a strange sound. It is a laugh. I can hardly believe it, for no one laughs on Thursday. Thursday is chemo day on 4B.

I scan the crowded reception area, looking for the source of the laughter. I note child after child, parent after parent. They all look the same—tired and frightened. I am certain each is thinking the same thought: Why is the treatment worse than the disease? My eyes lock on one particular mother who is holding her baby, a boy of about eight months. The laugh is his. He is bouncing on his mother's knee. It is obvious this is the child's favorite game. The mother's face is one big smile. She relishes the brief moments of happiness in her son's short life. She realizes it may be a while before he has the strength to smile again. He, too, has been chosen to suffer an unfair and uncertain fate. My eyes fill with tears.

I shift in my seat to get a better view of the baby. I stare at his small, bald head. Baldness is not unusual in an infant, but I know why he is hairless. Suddenly I become angry with myself. I despise it when people stare at me; however, here I am sharing the stares I abhor.

I shift my weight once again and sink more deeply into the groove of my chair. A rush of emotions—anger, fear, sadness, pity—surge through me. I remain deeply engrossed in my thoughts for a long time. A booming voice interrupts my reverie. It is the nurse summoning mother and baby into hell. Simultaneously the bouncing and laughing cease. The mother picks up her son. As they walk past me, I look at the baby once more. He is completely calm. His eyes are bright, and there is an expression of complete trust on his tiny face. I know that I will never forget that expression.

This is but one of many Thursdays. However, on this particular Thursday, many months into a seemingly endless series of treatments, I learned a lesson from a little baby. He changed my life. He taught me that anger, tears and sadness are only for those who have given up. He also taught me to trust. This I will carry with me always. Today, my little hero is doing fine. His last treatment is in sight and his future looks bright. I can honestly say that I am a little surprised. That bright-eyed baby appeared so pale and sick that day. However, that was before I learned to trust.

Everyone, some sooner than others, must endure his or her own personal "hell on earth." It is important to keep searching for the small joys, although they are sometimes the most elusive. Trust that these joys will appear, sometimes unexpectedly, and often in life's darkest moments . . . for instance, in the smile on a baby's face.

Katie Gill

Keep on Keeping On

In 1986, actress Jill Eikenberry completed the pilot for a new television show—*L.A. Law*. She and her husband, actor Michael Tucker, felt excited about the prospects for the show. They planned to leave their home in New York and move to Los Angeles if NBC accepted the pilot.

Suddenly their rosy future turned dark. In May, Eikenberry's doctor told her she had breast cancer.

"The news came completely out of the blue," Eikenberry told me. "At first, I thought that I was going to die and that was it. I spent some time just lying on the bed and crying, unable to imagine how my family was going to get along without me."

Husband Michael Tucker was scared, too. "I remember the moment when the doctor said, 'It's malignant.' I've never been so scared in my life. I thought I was going to lose her." But Tucker and Eikenberry gave each other strength. "Michael and I just held each other for a long time. That helped," Eikenberry says.

Then several days after learning the diagnosis, Eikenberry went to the screening of a film she'd recently done. One of the other actresses from the film was there, and when the young woman saw Eikenberry, she asked if something was wrong.

"I spilled it all out to her," Eikenberry says. "And she took me over to her mother who was there, too. When her mother heard the story, she grabbed me and dragged me into the ladies' room. She hiked up her blouse and said, 'Look, this is eleven years ago. I have a scar here and that's all I have to remind me of the breast cancer. This, too, can happen to you.'

"It was the first time I ever had any sense that there was hope, that I might not die," Eikenberry says. "Her words gave me the courage to seek a second opinion. The first doctor had told me a mastectomy was the best idea, but the second physician said no, I was a good candidate for a lumpectomy."

So Eikenberry opted to have the lumpectomy, a less radical procedure. The operation was successful, but treatment wasn't finished. When Eikenberry began filming the regular episodes of *L.A. Law*, she left the set every day at 3:30 P.M. to go to UCLA Medical Center for radiation treatment.

"She was exhausted," Tucker says. "After she got home, she'd rest for the rest of the night, and then go back to work the next day. And this is how we did the first three or four episodes of *L.A. Law*."

Eikenberry told me how it was for her. "I just had to keep on keeping on," she said. "And today everybody says, 'Oh, that must have been so hard for you.' And it was. But if you have something else you have to do, it helps. Continuing to work was very therapeutic. I was also playing the Ann Kelsey role, which was so strong and aggressive and confident. I think that really helped me make it through. Today, I'm celebrating my fifth anniversary cancer-free.

"Once you've fought something like cancer and won, there's not much that's scary. I used to be scared of flying, but I'm not anymore. After cancer, you've seen the thing that we all spend a lot of time denying. You've looked death in the face. So fear plays much less of a role in my life than it used to."

Jill Eikenberry kept on keeping on and discovered that change and setbacks really can make you stronger.

Erik Olesen

The Container

One of the angriest people I have ever worked with was a young man with osteogenic sarcoma of the right leg. He had been a high school and college athlete, and until the time of his diagnosis, his life had been good. Beautiful women, fast cars, personal recognition. Two weeks after his diagnosis, they had removed his right leg above the knee. This surgery, which saved his life, also ended his life. Playing ball was a thing of the past.

These days, there are many sorts of self-destructive behaviors open to an angry young man like this. He refused to return to school. He began to drink heavily, to use drugs, to alienate his former admirers and friends and to have one automobile accident after the other. After the second of these, his former coach called and referred him to me.

He was a powerfully built and handsome young man, profoundly self-oriented and isolated. At the beginning, he had the sort of rage that felt very familiar to me. Filled with a sense of injustice and self-pity, he hated all the well people. In our second meeting, hoping to encourage him to show his feelings about himself, I gave him a drawing pad and asked him to draw a picture of his body. He drew a crude sketch of a vase, just an outline. Running through the center of it he drew a deep crack. He went over and over the crack with a black crayon, gritting his teeth and tearing the paper. He had tears in his eyes. They were tears of rage. It seemed to me that the drawing was a powerful statement of his pain and the finality of his loss. It was clear that this broken vase could never hold water, could never function as a vase again. It hurt to watch. After he left, I folded the picture up and saved it. It seemed too important to throw away.

In time, his anger began to change in subtle ways. He began one session by handing me an item torn from our local newspaper. It was an article about a motorcycle accident in which a young man had lost his leg. His doctors were quoted at length. I finished reading and looked up. "Those idiots don't know the first thing about it," he said furiously. Over the next month he brought in more of these articles, some from the paper and some from magazines: a girl who had been severely burned in a house fire, a boy whose hand had been partly destroyed in the explosion of his chemistry set. His reactions were always the same, a harsh judgment of the well-meaning efforts of doctors and parents. His anger about these other young people began to occupy more and more of our session time. No one understood them, no one was there for them, no one really knew how to help them. He was still enraged, but it seemed to me that underneath this anger a concern for others was growing. Encouraged, I asked him if he wanted to do anything about it. Caught by surprise, at first he said, "No." But just before he left he asked me if I thought he could meet some of these others who suffered injuries like his.

People came to our hospital from all over the world, and the chances were good that there were some with the sorts of injuries that mattered to him. I said that I thought it was quite possible and I would look into it. It turned out to be easy. Within a few weeks, he had begun to visit young people on the surgical wards whose problems were similar to his own.

He came back from these visits full of stories, delighted to find that he could reach young people. He was often able to be of help when no one else could. After a while he felt able to speak to parents and families, helping them to better understand and to know what was needed. The surgeons, delighted with the results of these visits, referred more and more people to him. Some of these doctors had seen him play ball and they began to spend a little time with him. As he got to know them, his respect for them grew. Gradually his anger faded and he developed a sort of ministry. I just watched and listened and appreciated.

My favorite of all his stories concerned a visit to a young woman who had a tragic family history: breast cancer had claimed the lives of her mother, her sister and her cousin. Another sister was in chemotherapy. This last event had driven her into action. At 21 she had both her breasts removed surgically.

He visited her on a hot midsummer day, wearing shorts, his artificial leg in full view. Deeply depressed, she lay in bed with her eyes closed, refusing to look at him. He tried everything he knew to reach her but without success. He said things to her that only another person with an altered body would dare to say. He made jokes. He even got angry. She did not respond. All the while a radio was softly playing rock music. Frustrated, he finally stood, and in a last effort to get her attention he unstrapped the harness of his artificial leg and let it drop to the floor with a loud thump. Startled, she opened her eyes and saw him for the first time. This young man, once one of the best dancers on his college campus, began to hop around the room snapping his fingers in time to the music, laughing out loud at himself. After a moment she burst out laughing. "Fella," she said, "if you can dance, maybe I can sing."

This young woman became his friend and began to visit people in the hospital with him. She was in school and she encouraged him to return to school to study psychology and dream of carrying his work further. Eventually she became his wife, a very different sort of person from the models and cheerleaders he had dated in the past. But long before this, we ended our sessions together. In our final meeting, we were reviewing the way he had come, the sticking points and the turning points. I opened his chart and found the picture of the broken vase that he had drawn two years before. Unfolding it, I asked him if he remembered the drawing he had made of his body. He took it in his hands and looked at it for some time. "You know," he said, "it's really not finished." Surprised, I extended my basket of crayons toward him. Taking a yellow crayon, he began to draw lines radiating from the crack in the vase to the very edges of the paper. Thick yellow lines. I watched, puzzled. He was smiling. Finally he put his finger on the crack, looked at me and said softly, "This is where the light comes through."

Suffering is intimately connected to wholeness. The power in suffering to promote integrity is not only a Christian belief, it has been a part of almost every religious tradition. Yet 20 years of working with people with cancer, in the setting of unimaginable loss and pain, suggests that this may not be a spiritual teaching or a religious belief at all, but rather some sort of natural law. That is, we might learn it not by divine revelation, but simply through a careful and patient observation of the nature of the world. Suffering shapes the life force, some-times into anger, sometimes into blame and self-pity. Eventually it may show us the freedom of loving and serving life.

Rachel Naomi Remen, M.D.

3

ON ATTITUDE

It is our attitude at the beginning of a difficult undertaking which more than anything else, will determine its outcome.

William James

The Best Day of My Life

Today, when I awoke, I suddenly realized that this is the best day of my life, ever!

There were times when I wondered if I would make it to today; but I did! And because I did I'm going to celebrate!

Today, I'm going to celebrate what an unbelievable life I have had so far: the accomplishments, the many blessings, and, yes, even the hardships because they have served to make me stronger.

I will go through this day with my head held high and a happy heart. I will marvel at God's seemingly simple gifts: the morning dew, the sun, the clouds, the trees, the flowers, the birds. Today, none of these miraculous creations will escape my notice.

Today, I will share my excitement for life with other people. I'll make someone smile. I'll go out of my way to perform an unexpected act of kindness for someone I don't even know. Today, I'll give a sincere compliment to someone who seems down. I'll tell a child how special he is, and I'll tell someone I love just how deeply I care for her and how much she means to me.

Today is the day I quit worrying about what I don't have and start being grateful for all the wonderful things God has already given me. I'll remember that to worry is just a waste of time because my faith in God and his Divine Plan ensures everything will be just fine.

And tonight, before I go to bed, I'll go outside and raise my eyes to the heavens. I will stand in awe at the beauty of the stars and the moon, and I will praise God for these magnificent treasures.

As the day ends and I lay my head down on my pillow, I will thank the Almighty for the best day of my life. And I will sleep the sleep of a contented child, excited with expectation because I know tomorrow is going to be the best day of my life, ever!

Gregory M. Lousig-Nont, Ph.D.

Love Is Stronger . . .

Having a goal based on love is the greatest life insurance in the world.

If you had asked my dad why he got up in the morning, you would have found his answer disarmingly simple: "To make my wife happy."

Mom and Dad met when they were nine. Every day before school, they met on a park bench with their homework. Mom corrected Dad's English and he did the same with her math. Upon graduation, their teachers said that the two of them were the best "student" in the school. Note the singular!

They took their time building their relationship, even though Dad always knew she was the girl for him. Their first kiss occurred when they were 17, and their romance continued to grow into their 80s.

Just how much power their relationship created was brought to light in 1964. The doctor told Dad he had cancer and estimated that he had six months to one year left at the most.

"Sorry to disagree with you, Doc," my father said. "But I'll tell you how long I have. One day longer than my wife.

I love her too much to leave the planet without her."

And so it was, to the amazement of everyone who didn't really know this love-matched pair, that Mom passed away at the age of 85 and Dad followed one year later when he was 86. Near the end, he told my brothers and me that those 17 years were the best six months he ever spent.

To the wonderful doctors and nurses at the Department of Veterans' Affairs Medical Center at Long Beach, he was a walking miracle. They kept a loving watch on him and just couldn't understand how a body so riddled with cancer could continue to function so well.

My dad's explanation was simple. He informed them that he had been a medic in World War I and saw amputated arms and legs, and he had noticed that none of them could think. So he decided he would tell his body how to behave. Once, as he stood up and it was evident he felt a stabbing pain, he looked down at his chest and shouted, "Shut up! We're having a party here."

Two days before he left us he said, "Boys, I'll be with your mother very soon and someday, some place we'll all be together again. But take your time about joining us; your mother and I have a lot of catching up to do."

It is said that love is stronger than prison walls. Dad proved it was a heck of a lot stronger than tiny cancer cells.

Bob, George and I are still here, armed with Dad's final gift.

A goal, a love and a dream give you total control over your body and your life.

John Wayne Schlatter

The Power to Choose

When one door of happiness closes, another opens; but often we look so long at the closed door that we do not see the one which has opened for us.

Helen Keller

I always feel good when I'm in Angela Passidomo Trafford's office. I feel validated, nurtured and somehow better about myself. On this occasion I was there to talk about the workshop she was co-facilitating that month with well-known author and surgeon, Bernie Siegel, M.D.

When I asked how she chose the title of the workshop, "The Power to Choose," Angela explained, "Most people are paralyzed in their ability to make a decision and in their ability to choose. They are paralyzed with their conditioning of the past and with the guilt and shame of the past."

Angela speaks from personal experience. As told in her book, *The Heroic Path*, she recalled to me the low point of her life that led her to Bernie's book. She hit rock bottom after finding out on the same day that she lost custody of her children and that she had cancer. "I fell on my knees and let go of my life to God. I asked God to take my life and show me how to live because I realized that I did not know how.

"Afterward, I found myself just wandering through the public library; I didn't even know what I was doing there. The librarian came up to me—I didn't even know her—and she had Bernie Siegel's book, Love, Medicine and Miracles, in her hand. She asked me if I had read it. When I shook my head no, she said, 'Well, you should!' That was the beginning of what I referred to often as a divine plan, how one thing leads to another and puts you in touch with the idea that there is a plan for your life. Getting in touch with that connection to a higher intelligence inside each and every one of us, that's what healing and life are all about.

"My divine plan continued unfolding when I took Bernie Siegel's book home and found this eminent surgeon saying things that I had felt all my life. He had put forth this whole philosophy of taking charge of your life, and taking charge of your health and being responsible for your feelings. And going within to heal.

"I began waking up early in the morning and giving thanks for the gift of life. I realized that even though everything had been taken from me, I still had this amazing awareness that life itself is a great gift, and I felt tremendous gratitude for that gift.

"I would ride my bike and then go home and do the meditation and visualization exercises outlined in the book. One day a visualization came forth from a creative source. I visualized these little birds eating golden crumbs; the little birds were the immune system cells and the golden crumbs the cancer cells. I followed this visualization by imagining a white light coming through the top of my head, flowing through my body, healing me.

"During the three weeks before my scheduled surgical biopsy, I continued meditating each morning after my bike ride, until one morning, all of a sudden I felt this tremendous, powerful white light coursing through my body. I was alarmed and my rational mind screamed in all its conditioning of fear and mistrust, 'Get out, get out, you're having a heart attack, stop the experience.' But I chose to let go and allow my being to become one with the beautiful light, that powerful energy.

"Afterward I just slumped over on the couch. And for the first time in my life I had no thoughts at all. Just this tremendous feeling of peace. And I knew something wonderful had happened to me.

"My next visit to the doctor's confirmed what I already knew. The cancer had disappeared.

"This experience changed my life. I began a mission to share my experience with others facing the illness of cancer. Lots has happened since then. I acquired the custody of my children, opened my business, Self Healing, and wrote my first book, *The Heroic Path*, describing my journey from cancer to self-healing.

"I believe this is a time in our world that people are awakening to the possibility of more joy in our lives. The universe offers us endless opportunities to let go of the fear and the guilt and the shame and the anger, all the repressed issues of the past.

"Health is a choice. We choose to be healthy, we choose joy, we choose happiness. These are all choices that we make when we have the power to choose. But in order to feel that power, we have to learn what it means to love ourselves and be empowered as individuals—and I have discovered how to do that in day-to-day life."

Sharon Bruckman

Laugh!

Many years ago, Norman Cousins was diagnosed as "terminally ill." He was given six months to live. His chance for recovery was one in 500.

He could see that the worry, depression and anger in his life contributed to, and perhaps helped cause, his disease. He wondered, "If illness can be caused by negativity, can wellness be created by positivity?"

He decided to make an experiment of himself. Laughter was one of the most positive activities he knew. He rented all the funny movies he could find—Keaton, Chaplin, Fields, the Marx Brothers. (This was before VCRs, so he had to rent the actual films.) He read funny stories. He asked his friends to call him whenever they said, heard or did something funny.

His pain was so great he could not sleep. Laughing for 10 solid minutes, he found, relieved the pain for several hours so he could sleep.

He fully recovered from his illness and lived another 20 happy, healthy and productive years. (His journey is detailed in his book, *Anatomy of an Illness.*) He credits visualization, the love of his family and friends, and laughter for his recovery.

Some people think laughter is a waste of time. It is a luxury, they say, a frivolity, something to indulge in only every so often.

Nothing could be further from the truth. Laughter is essential to our equilibrium, to our well-being, to our aliveness. If we're not well, laughter helps us get well; if we are well, laughter helps us stay that way.

Since Cousins' ground-breaking subjective work, scientific studies have shown that laughter has a curative effect on the body, the mind and the emotions.

So, if you like laughter, consider it sound medical advice to indulge in it as often as you can. If you don't like laughter, then take your medicine—laugh anyway.

Use whatever makes you laugh—movies, sitcoms, Monty Python, records, books, *New Yorker* cartoons, jokes, friends.

Give yourself permission to laugh—long and loud and out loud—whenever anything strikes you as funny. The people around you may think you're strange, but sooner or later they'll join in even if they don't know what you're laughing about.

Some diseases may be contagious, but none is as contagious as the cure . . . laughter.

Peter McWilliams

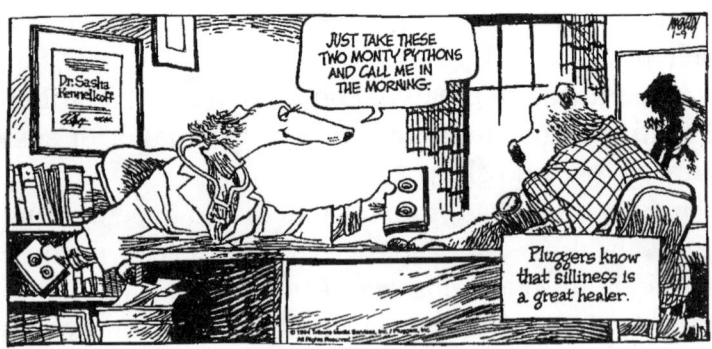

Reprinted by permission: Tribune Media Services.

The "Wee" Nurse

There ain't much fun in medicine, but there's a heck of a lot of medicine in fun.

Josh Billings

When I was in the hospital, I had a "We" nurse. She began each sentence with "How are we today?" "We need to have a bath." This really irritated me, so I decided to play a little joke on her.

One day, she brought in a specimen cup and requested a urine sample. After she left, I poured my apple juice into the cup. When she returned for the specimen, she observed it and noted, "My, we're a little cloudy today, aren't we?"

I asked to see it, removed the lid and said, "Yep, better run it through again," and drank it. The look of shock on her face was priceless.

Norman Cousins

Until Tomorrow Comes

*The tragedy of life is not that it ends so soon,
but that we wait so long to begin it.*

Anonymous

Our lives changed drastically on a spring day that
started like any other—in a humdrum way. The alarm
clock rang, I dressed quickly and headed downstairs to
make breakfast for my husband, Orville, and our four
children.

In the kitchen I set the table, put the coffeepot on the
stove to perk and prepared oatmeal. The sun was just
coming up, and it was probably a glorious sight rising
over the Mississippi (we can see the river from our house),
but I was too preoccupied to notice. I was still trying to
figure out the math problem that had stumped my 13-
year-old son, Mark, and me the night before.

Before I could solve the problem, Orville interrupted
my thoughts by slumping into his chair at the table.
"Honey," he said with a sigh, "I discovered something
just now as I was washing under my arm—I felt a lump
there."

Even though our kitchen was toasty warm, a chill of fear swept through my body as I recalled how Orville had been coming home from work for months complaining of being so tired. But I didn't want anything serious to touch this husky man I loved so much, so I said, "Now, don't worry so much. You're probably still feeling the effects of that flu you've had. But if the lump doesn't go away in a few days, you should have it checked."

By the time he went to the doctor several days later, there were three lumps. Orville told him about the nagging tired feeling and his lack of energy.

"Well, we'll remove one of the lumps," the doctor said matter-of-factly, "and have it checked."

When the day came for the biopsy, we took my mother and Mark with us to the hospital. I didn't say anything to Tammy, 11, Lori, 8, or Britt, 4, about their father's problem. While waiting in the hospital lounge, my mother and I passed the time by recounting events of the 14 years since Orville and I had married. There was our first meeting one morning in the little restaurant where I worked—Orville's big brown eyes were heart-melters—marriage, children, chicken pox, drafty farmhouses, overdue fuel bills, Orville's struggle to find his calling. He had made a lot of job changes before he began writing for newspapers—and then his search was over. He loved newspaper work.

We kept talking about our lives until Mark interrupted us. I looked up to see a nurse beckoning; she escorted me into an office. The doctor was mercifully quick. "Mrs. Kelly, your husband has lymphoma."

"Can-cer?" I stammered. I could hardly bring myself to say the word. Numbly I stumbled out of the doctor's office. My eyes burned and I knew I was about to cry, but I bit my lip and drove a fingernail into my palm. "Not here, Wanda, not here," I told myself.

Straightening, I marched down the hall to the office to see about Blue Cross and hospital papers, then to the lobby and outside. The cold air had barely hit my face when the first tear ran down my cheek. By the time I got to the parking lot I was sobbing uncontrollably. "Mom, I'm going to lose him," I wailed. "Why, God? He's only 42."

After a couple of minutes I pulled myself together, dried my eyes, powdered my face and pasted on a smile. By the time we drove around to the hospital entrance to pick up Orville, I thought I looked okay, but he knew I'd been crying. "Don't worry, honey," he said as he stepped into the car. "I'll be all right." But his voice was listless, and I had to clench my teeth to keep from crying again.

After dropping off Orville, Mark and Mother at the house, I took the babysitter home. Hurrying back to my family, I passed a church and suddenly decided to go in. I was grateful there was no one there because I ran down the aisle and threw myself on the floor in front of the altar.

"God, dear God," I sobbed, "please give us a miracle. Heal Orville. I beg You." I don't know how long I lay there pleading, weeping, but after a while I got up, left the church and went on home.

Orville was lying on the davenport, staring at the ceiling. We exchanged some meaningless conversation and I went to the kitchen to fix dinner. At the table the kids were as noisy as ever, but Orville ate in silence and left as soon as he was finished. Not once did he say anything about the doctor's report and not once did the word cancer come up in our conversation.

After further hospital tests, the doctors told Orville he might have as little as six months or as long as three years to live.

From then on, Orville and I talked very little to each other. A tension built up in our home. The gaiety that had always been a part of our marriage and our household was gone. No longer were there picnics or barbecues or rides for an evening ice cream cone, as we commonly did in the past.

Although the children didn't know what was wrong, they became edgy and upset. I was sometimes sharp with Mother, and she cried over the slightest thing. When I tried to talk to friends about our situation, they said, "Don't think about it," and tried to change the subject. Gradually, perhaps out of fear and not knowing what to say, our friends stopped seeing us. There was no one to talk to, nothing to say. I've never felt so alone or lonely in my life. And I knew it was even worse for Orville.

He spent most of his time in the study lying down. In fact, he slept there at night. Coming to bed with me would have meant that we had to talk to each other, something neither of us could bear. Though I wanted to say something loving, positive, hopeful, and I was sure he wanted to reassure me, we couldn't find any honest words, so we remained silent.

Meanwhile, I spent hours pleading with God. And every night before going to bed I prayed the same prayer. "God, heal Orville, please. . . . "

Then Orville was placed on chemotherapy. For his treatments, we drove to a hospital in Iowa City. I'll never forget that first return trip. We had taken Britt along and he was asleep in the back seat. Inside the car we rode in complete silence except for the purr of the engine and the humming of the tires.

Suddenly Orville spoke, clearly and distinctly, in a tone I hadn't heard for weeks. "Wanda," he said, "you know, I'm not dead yet." Abruptly he pulled the car off the highway and parked. "Honey, I've got cancer. Cancer. And I'll probably die of it. But I'm not dead yet. We've got to talk about it."

I reached over and touched his hand. "Are you sure you want to?"

"Yes, I'm sure," he continued. "We've got to face it together. I know you haven't told me the way you really feel. I don't know how we can help each other if we don't talk about it. I've just been moping around the house making everyone miserable." He took a deep breath. "Let's go home and have a barbecue tonight," he said. "And tell the kids. I don't want to waste any more time living like we have."

Pulling me to him, Orville threw his arms around me and gave me a long kiss. For the first time in weeks I felt a flicker of our old happiness. The sun was shining brilliantly on the rich fields and bright fall leaves. Part of a great burden had been lifted off my shoulders and I felt alive again.

I bought spareribs on the way home and that evening we cooked out, just like old times. After dinner I put little Britt to bed and we called Mark, Tammy and Lori to join us on the back porch.

It was a lovely starlit night. In the distance the moon shimmered on the Mississippi. As the children gathered around, Orville said, "I think it's time you knew what's wrong with me." Then he explained that he had cancer— a disease that destroys parts of the body—and the doctors said he would probably die of it. Tammy's eyes filled with tears and Orville drew her to him.

"But I'm not dead yet, honey. I've started treatments and I'm going to stay alive just as long as I possibly can. Sometimes things may get bad, but I want you all to help me to live with this. We don't have to like death, but we don't have to be terrified by it either."

Orville hugged and kissed each child and saw them off to bed. As he did, a dark cloud seemed to lift from our house. After the children left, Orville and I sat together on the porch for a long time.

"Wanda," he finally said, taking my hand, "when this happened, I cursed God. Why did He do this to me?

Why not somebody like that drunk down the street who has no family?"

"Well, driving home from the hospital today in our deathly silent car, I felt so bad I finally turned to God for an answer. And do you know what my answer was? To go home and barbecue. To start living again. Why not? I thought. I can still move about. The very idea that almost normal life could go on, if I'd allow it, really charged me up."

Orville turned and put his arm around me. "You know, honey, it's like being on a train, and far ahead of you down the track you see your final destination. But there are many station stops in between. Well, instead of concentrating on that final destination, I decided to take advantage of each stop along the way and make the most of the remainder of the journey.

"Wanda, I don't really know how many days I have left. For that matter, none of us knows how much time we have left on this earth. So why not grab each day as it comes, make the most of it, explore it to the fullest, enjoy all its delights and treasures."

With his new attitude, new energy seemed to flow into Orville. A few days later he sat down at his typewriter and wrote an article for the Burlington newspaper, telling how it feels to be a person with a terminal illness. After the story appeared, we were deluged with letters from all kinds of patients and their families. It gave Orville the idea of starting some kind of club. Maybe people in life-threatening situations could help one another. The first meeting was held on January 25, 1974, in the Burlington Elks lodge. The 18 people who attended decided to call their group Make Today Count (MTC). Others heard of MTC and formed chapters around the country. Soon Orville was traveling all over the country, speaking and giving interviews.

And my life changed, too. As I grew more aware of the potential of each and every day, I gained the incentive to finish high school. Last year, realizing that I might someday shoulder responsibility for our family's welfare, I completed my high school credits. Later on I hope to go to college.

Even more important, as I've watched Orville renew himself, my own faith in God has blossomed. God had always been real to me, but now, being involved in something so positive and fulfilling as MTC, I'm discovering new strength in God and feel that His word comforts me more than ever.

The other day Orville drew my attention to the lilacs outside our door. They were full-budded, waiting to break forth once more. They reminded me so much of Orville's own renewal.

Orville Kelly's Ten Suggestions:

1. Talk about the illness. If it is cancer, call it cancer. You can't make life normal again by trying to hide what is wrong.
2. Accept death as a part of life. It is.
3. Consider each day as another day of life, a gift from God to be enjoyed as fully as possible.
4. Realize that life is never going to be perfect. It wasn't before and it won't be now.
5. Pray. It isn't a sign of weakness; it is your strength.
6. Learn to live with your illness instead of considering yourself dying from it. We are all dying in some manner.
7. Put your friends and relatives at ease yourself. If you don't want pity, don't ask for it.
8. Make all practical arrangements for funerals, wills, etc., and make certain your family understands them.

9. Set new goals; realize your limitations. Sometimes the simple things of life become the most enjoyable.
10. Discuss your problems with your family as they occur. Include the children if possible. After all, your problem is not an individual one.

Wanda Kelly

EDITOR'S NOTE: In his recent book, *Make Today Count* (Delacorte Press), Orville Kelly tells how the organization that bears the same name helps terminally ill people cope with their problems. Says Kelly of MTC meetings, "They give cancer patients an opportunity to talk honestly about their feelings and to discuss their anxieties and fears with others whose circumstances are similar." In addition to informal discussions, ministers, psychiatrists, physicians and lawyers are often asked to speak at meetings. There are now some 60 MTC chapters around the country.

If you would like to know how you can help, or if you want additional information about Make Today Count, please write to: Make Today Count, Mid-America Cancer Center, 1235 E. Cherokee, Springfield, MO 65804, or call 800-432-2273.

Two Things Not to Worry About

In my life, I have found there are two things about which I should never worry. First, I shouldn't worry about the things I can't change. If I can't change them, worry is certainly most foolish and useless. Second, I shouldn't worry about the things I can change. If I can change them, then taking action will accomplish far more than wasting my energies in worry. Besides, it is my belief that, 9 times out of 10, worrying about something does more danger than the thing itself. Give worry its rightful place—out of your life.

Source Unknown

Head First

The greatest discovery of any generation is that human beings can alter their lives by altering the attitudes of their minds.

Albert Schweitzer

Perhaps the most striking experience of all came late in 1978, just as Ellen and I were about to leave for China. A physician in Sherman Oaks telephoned and identified himself as Dr. Avrum Bluming. He was calling about his patient, a judge, who was in the terminal stage of cancer and who was then at the Encino Hospital. He said the judge's mood was understandably bleak. All of his personal and professional life he had been known for courage, determination and a positive outlook on life. His illness, however, had given him the psychology of fatalism. He told his wife and children that there was no hope and that he expected to die very soon.

Dr. Bluming told me that the effect of the judge's mood on the family was catastrophic. He said that the judge's seeming willingness to give up without a fight was totally out of character. The physician was worried that the judge's wife might be vulnerable to serious illness.

On the way to the airport for the flight to China, I stopped off at the Encino Hospital. Before entering the judge's room, I met with Dr. Bluming, who told me that the judge had virtually stopped eating and was resisting intravenous feeding. At the present rate, he said, it was doubtful that he would survive more than two or three days.

When I entered the room, the judge made me sit close to the bedside. He spoke in a hoarse whisper and it was difficult to follow what he was saying, but I picked up enough to learn that he had been a longtime reader of the *Saturday Review* and had sympathetically followed its various enthusiasms and concerns.

I took his hand and thanked him and told him that few things in my life were more gratifying than to meet readers of the magazine. I asked how he felt. He closed his eyes and shook his head.

I said that Dr. Bluming had given me a briefing on his condition and that I was also concerned about his wife and sons and, in fact, about all the people who loved him.

His eyes narrowed in a way that indicated he wanted me to explain myself. I said I understood that all his life he had been a fighter for things he considered just and right.

He nodded and again he narrowed his eyes, as though to find out what I was getting at.

I said that one of the things I had learned at the medical school was that the attitude of the patient had a profound effect on members of the family. Their health could be jeopardized by the negative attitude of the patient. I said that I hoped he would forgive me if I said that his family was anguished by the judge's apparent defeatism. Such defeatism might seem natural in anyone else, but in the judge . . .

The judge closed his eyes momentarily. Then he looked at me and uttered just two words: "I gotcha."

The emphasis and sense of purpose even in his whisper

were unmistakable, as was the pressure of his handshake before I left.

When Ellen and I arrived in Hong Kong, the first thing I did was to telephone the Encino Hospital. Dr. Bluming went out to the nurse's station to take the call.

"Something is happening here that you'll find difficult to believe," he said. "When the nurse began to rig up the intravenous device, the judge demanded that he be given breakfast on a tray. This was done. He got the food down, and kept it down. How he did that I'll never know. When his wife arrived, he called her to the bedside, then invited her to work on problems that come up in bridge games. The judge used to be a tournament bridge player. Where he got the energy to concentrate on bridge, I have no idea.

"This isn't all," he continued. "After bridge, he asked for a robe and slippers, he got out of bed, and went to the bathroom on his own. When the nurse tried to restrain him, saying she wanted him to use the bedpan, he waved her off and said he could take care of himself. He was crusty and strong-willed—just the way people had always known him."

I asked if this was any indication that the underlying situation had changed.

"Not so far as I can tell, but it sure has made a difference in the lives of his wife and children. He's going to survive this weekend and then some."

After I arrived in China, we were escorted into the interior of the country where international telephone facilities were not readily available. It was not until two weeks later, when we arrived in Shanghai, that I was able to telephone the hospital again.

This time, the judge's wife went out to the nurse's station to take the call. Her voice was strong and cheerful.

"The judge's spirits have been wonderful," she said. "He

has had good talks with our sons. He follows the newspapers and makes his usual witty comments. Now he takes walks in the hospital corridors and chats with other patients. The ultimate outlook hasn't changed, but the general atmosphere has. We are ... well, a lot less despondent than we were."

The judge survived for several more weeks. It was a magnificent example of how the human spirit could make a difference—not just in prolonging one's life, but in bolstering the lives of others. The judge's deep sense of purpose didn't reverse the disease—the cancer had spread so widely to his vital organs that it was only a question of time before it would claim his life. But he was able to prolong his life beyond the expectations of the physician. He was also able to govern the circumstances of his passing in a way that provided spiritual nourishment to the people who loved him. He died in character. This was his gift to everyone who knew him.

Norman Cousins

I've Just Got to Make That Man Laugh!

In order to laugh, you must be able to play with your pain.

Annette Goodheart

Bobby was 13, one of nine kids in his Portuguese-American family, with beautiful, thick, silky black hair and liquid expressive eyes. A quiet boy, a polite boy, loved by his teachers and worshipped by his younger brothers and sisters.

His family were milkers, living and working on another family's ranch, eking out their living and taking care of the cows. A loving but strictly religious family, they rose early and worked hard every day just to make ends meet.

It was a disaster beyond expression when Bobby was diagnosed with leukemia and later with bone cancer. His parents struggled to contain their grief, worry and fear. His father hid his pain behind a screen of stoicism and unrelenting work. His mother seemed to walk through each day with tears hiding just behind her eyes.

They did their chores, then took Bobby in for his

treatments, enduring the costs of time, money and uncertainty as best they could. Their love for Bobby was expressed without drama or display, in those silent looks shared when they didn't think he'd notice and in their bluff assertions to him that they knew he'd recover from this "cancer thing." It never occurred to them that humor was missing from their lives, so deeply were they enmeshed in the struggle for economic survival and the physical survival of their eldest son. Every morning and evening, the clockwork of their lives turned and it was time for milking. Now added to these chiming hours were the regular medications and treatments for their boy.

Near the end of Bobby's struggle with his disease, he told me this story.

"When I was admitted to the hospital for the first long series of treatments, there was a male nurse, Floyd, who reminded me of a middle linebacker. He was huge and never seemed to smile.

"Floyd came into my room one day with the breathing machine. Because I was too weak to do much other than lie in bed, my lungs were affected. He told me that I had to use this breathing machine and puff into it repeatedly. It had some little plastic ball that had to be puffed up to a certain mark on the machine. He had attached a little figurine of a hula dancer to the end of the machine's air pipe. 'Okay, kid,' he said, 'If you really puff hard, you'll lift the hula dancer's grass skirt!' And without a smile, he left the room.

"I was amazed at what he said and that a nurse would do such a crazy thing. But I had to laugh. And I sure had to try to puff that skirt up! I ended up doing that machine so much they had to take it away from me for a while! That hula dancer helped a lot. And I laughed and laughed. I showed it to my brothers, too. But I couldn't let my parents know because my mother and father would have been shocked.

"Then, one day, I was told about the radiation treatments and the chemotherapy I would have to go through. As the treatments progressed, my hair began falling out. When Floyd wheeled me back to my room after one grueling session, he brought in a paper bag and took out from it an atrocious, ugly, wild, black wig and a lollipop. He put this ill-fitting wig on his head and sucked on the lollipop as he said, 'You have a choice, kid. It's the rug or Kojak. You can get a wig, but you've got to know what people look like wearing one, or you can go with the bald head, but then you've got to suck on lollipops, like the TV star.' With that, he deposited the wig and a fresh sucker on my lap and walked out of the room. I began laughing and laughed so hard I couldn't stop myself. He had taken what seemed so horrible and made it so funny that I could live with it. It didn't seem to matter after that whether I had hair or not. I just kept picturing that big man in his green surgical scrubs and the ugly wig. If he could look like that, I could, too."

Today, Bobby is a thriving teenager with pimples, a patched-together pickup truck made from his uncle's hand-me-downs and assorted parts found in junkyards. He's got a girlfriend and the most upbeat attitude of any kid in town. These are the simple pleasures of his age.

Floyd introduced him to a tool that he could use for a lifetime of pleasures—the hopefulness of looking for the lighter, brighter, unexpected side of even the hardest times.

Meladee and Hanoch McCarty

The Prosthesis Intruder

Nothing is quite as funny as the unintended humor of reality.

Steve Allen

I am not usually the self-conscious type, even though I had my leg amputated when I was 10 due to cancer.

I believe that not only has growing up with just one leg not stunted my outdoor physical prowess, it has actually accelerated my love of snorkeling, dancing and hiking. Also, living with one leg has provided for quite a few humorous situations, like the following:

"Dave, wake up! Dave! Somebody's down in the basement!"

I couldn't for the life of me wake up Dave. I heard a noise like someone stumbling around drunk in our basement! Since it was quite apparent my heavy-sleeper hubby, Dave, was not going to be inconvenienced by this pesky intruder, I called the police.

I answered the door in my wheelchair and told the police where I believed the noises were coming from. Two of the officers went out to the backyard to check for footprints in the light powder snow we had in March, and the other officer went down into the basement to check for a prowler.

A few minutes later the two officers from outside came in and said they saw no footprints, and we waited for the other officer to return from the basement. Well, when he did return from the basement he was breathing heavily and ashen-faced.

We knew he must have come face to face with this intruder who left no footprints in the snow. We waited for him to catch his breath and he said in a gasping voice, "You didn't tell me about the artificial legs in the basement!" (I did answer the door in a wheelchair!)

It turns out that while he was cautiously surveying the basement, he came upon one of my shoed legs sticking out of the closet. He claims he "drew his gun and almost shot the darned thing!"

Needless to say, after we all stopped laughing hysterically at 2 A.M. and the poor guy stopped quivering, they told me that this was the most interesting night-shift call to tell their fellow officers.

Well, men in blue, happy to be of service.

Maureen J. Khan-Lacoss

The Value of Laughter

I had gone to the hospital because a group of doctors there were concerned that the mood of the cancer patients was so bleak, they feared the collective environment of treatment was being impaired.

At the suggestion of the doctors, I met with the veterans in the cancer unit. There were perhaps 50 or 60 of them. They sat in rows and were every bit as glum as I had anticipated.

I reported my conversation to their doctors, and said I doubted that they were helping them or themselves with the grim mood of the place. Certainly one could understand the reason for their feelings—and it was arrogant for anyone to lecture to them about it. But in coming to Sepulveda Veterans, they were reaching out for help—and they were entitled to know what would optimize that prospect.

I told them any battle with serious illness involved two elements. One was represented by the ability of the physicians to make available to patients the best that medical science has to offer. The other element was represented by the ability of patients to summon all their physical and spiritual resources in fighting illness.

I said I hoped the veterans would agree that their part of the job was to create an environment in which the doctors could do their best. One thing they might do to replace the grim atmosphere was to put on performances. We could give them scripts of amusing one-act plays. Some of them might wish to produce or direct or act. If they wished, we could help them obtain videocassettes of amusing motion picture films. Ditto, audiocassettes of stand-up comics. One way or another, their part in the joint enterprise with their doctors was to create a mood conducive to the best medical treatment obtainable.

The veterans accepted the challenge. When I returned to the hospital several weeks later and spoke to the doctors, I was pleased to have them describe the change not just in the general environment but in the mood of the individual patients.

When I met with the veterans, they no longer sat in a row. They sat in a large circle. They were part of a unity; they could all see one another. When they began their meeting, each veteran was obligated to tell something good that had happened to him since the previous meeting.

The first veteran spoke of his success in reaching by telephone a buddy he had not seen since the Korean War. He had tracked his buddy to Chicago and finally made the connection. They spoke for a half-hour or more. And the good news was that his buddy was coming to visit him in California.

Cheers.

The next veteran read from a letter he had received from a nephew who had just been admitted to medical school. He quoted the final sentence of the letter:

"And, Uncle Ben, I want you to know that I'm going into cancer research, and I'm going to come up with the answer, so you and your buddies just hang in there until I do."

More cheers.

And so it went, each person at the meeting taking his turn. Then I discovered that everyone was looking at me and that I was expected to report on what it was that was good that had happened to me.

I searched my recent memory and realized that something quite good had in fact happened to me only a few days earlier.

"What I have to report is better than good," I said. "It's wonderful. Actually, it's better than wonderful. It's unbelievable. And as long as I live, I don't expect that anything as magnificent as this can possibly happen to me again."

The veterans sat forward in their seats.

"What happened is that when I arrived at the Los Angeles airport last Wednesday, my bag was the first off the carousel."

An eruption of applause and acclaim greeted this announcement.

"I had never even met anyone whose bag was the first off the carousel," I continued.

Again, loud expressions of delight.

"Flushed with success, I went to the nearest telephone to report my arrival to my office. That was when I lost my coin. I pondered this melancholy event for a moment or two, then decided to report it to the operator.

" 'Operator,' I said, 'I put in a quarter and didn't get my number. The machine collected my coin.'

" 'Sir,' she said, 'if you give me your name and address, we'll mail the coin to you.'

"I was appalled.

" 'Operator, I said, 'I think I can understand the reason behind the difficulties of AT&T. You're going to take the time and trouble to write down my name on a card and then you are probably going to give it to the person in charge of such matters. He will go to the cash register, punch it open and take out a quarter, at the same time recording the reason for the cash withdrawal. Then he will take a cardboard with a recessed slot to hold the coin so it won't flop around in the envelope. Then he, or someone else, will fit the cardboard with the coin into an envelope, first taking the time to write out my address on the envelope. Then the envelope will be sealed. Someone will then affix a first-class stamp on the envelope. All that time and expense just to return a quarter. Now, operator, why don't you just return my coin and let's be friends.'

" 'Sir,' she repeated in a flat voice, 'if you give me your name and address, we will mail you the refund.'

"Then, almost by way of afterthought, she said, 'Sir, did you remember to press the coin return plunger?'

"Truth to tell, I had overlooked this nicety. I pressed the plunger. To my great surprise, it worked. It was apparent that the machine had been badly constipated and I happened to have the plunger. All at once, the vitals of the machine opened up and proceeded to spew out coins of almost every denomination. The profusion was so great that I had to use my empty hand to contain the overflow.

"While all this was happening, the noise was registering in the telephone and was not lost on the operator.

" 'Sir,' she said, 'what is happening?'

"I reported that the machine had just given up all its earnings for the past few months, at least. At a rough estimate, I said there must be close to four dollars in quarters, dimes and nickels that had just erupted from the box.

" 'Sir,' she said, 'will you please put the coins back in the box.'

" 'Operator,' I said, 'if you give me your name and address, I will be glad to mail you the coins.' "

The veterans exploded with cheers. David triumphs over Goliath. At the bottom of the ninth inning, with the home team behind by three runs, the weakest hitter in the lineup hits the ball out of the park. A mammoth business corporation is brought to its knees. Every person who had been exasperated by the loss of a coin in a public telephone booth could identify with my experience and share both in the triumph of justice and the humiliation of the mammoth and impersonal oppressor.

The veterans not only were having a good time; they were showing it in their relaxed expressions and in the way they moved.

One of the doctors stood up.

"Tell me," he said, "how many of you, when you came into this room a half hour or so ago, were experiencing, more or less, your normal chronic pains?"

More than half the veterans in the room raised their hands.

"Now," said the doctor, "how many of you in the past five or ten minutes discovered that these chronic pains receded or disappeared?"

The same hands, it appeared to me, went up again.

Why should simple laughter have produced this effect? Brain researchers with whom I have spoken have speculated that the laughter activated the release of endorphins, the body's own pain-reducing substance. The veterans were experiencing the same effects that had occurred to me in my own bout with inflammatory joints many years earlier. The body's own morphine was at work.

In view of what is now known about the role of endorphins not only as a painkiller but as a stimulant to the immune system, the biological value of laughter takes on scientific validity.

"If you wish to glimpse inside a human soul and get to know a man," Dostoevski writes in his novel, *The Adolescent*, "don't bother analyzing his ways of being silent, of talking, of weeping, or seeing how much he is moved by noble ideas; you'll get better results if you just watch him laugh. If he laughs well, he's a good man."

Norman Cousins

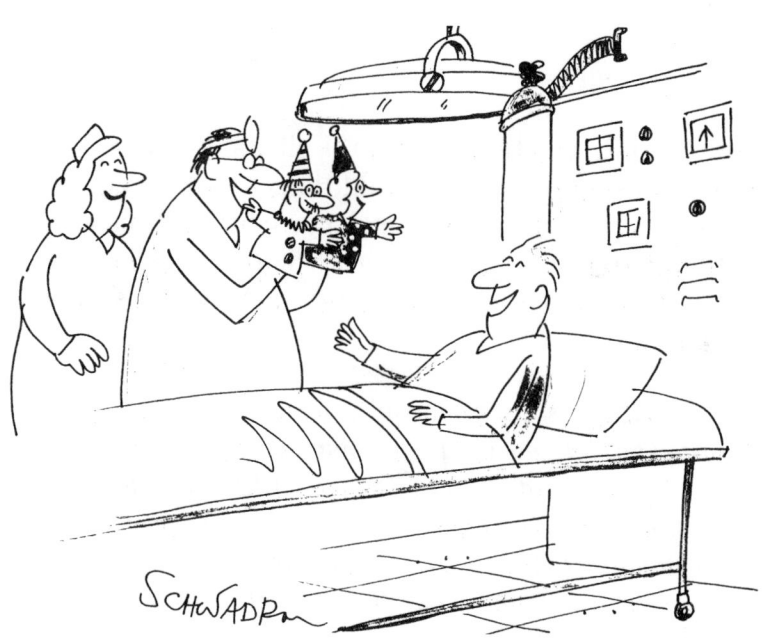

"It's a new surgical approach. We keep you in stitches so we won't have to sew you up afterwards."

Reprinted with permission from Harley Schwadron.

Second Thoughts

He who laughs, lasts.

Mary Pettibone Poole

In his introduction to Dan Keller's book *Humor as Therapy*, psychotherapist Gerald Piaget writes about how a juxtaposition of a humorous comment and his client's contemplation of suicide actually helped his client have second thoughts about taking her own life. His patient, Carol, told him:

> *Well, I was feeling horrible. You were gone, my husband was in no mood to hear more bitching, and I was really depressed. So I called Joan [Piaget's wife and Carol's best friend] to talk. During our conversation, I mentioned that with the cancer, and the depression, and the uncertainty and all, maybe there was no use even going on.*
>
> *I said it sort of casually, but in truth thoughts of suicide had been coming up for a couple of days. Now, Joan knows I'm not the suicidal type, but she got really angry at me.*

"Damn it, Carol!" she yelled. "If you dare kill yourself I swear to Christ I'll go to that cemetery and piss all over your grave!"

That image hasn't worn off, at least not yet. You know this hasn't been a very good week for me. But whenever I think of killing myself, I get this ridiculous image of Joan out there in the graveyard, with her eyes angry and her lower lip stuck out and her skirt hiked up around her waist, just squatting there on my grave. . . . It lightens me up, and I just don't feel like dying anymore. . . .

Allen Klein
from The Healing Power of Humor

Having an Attitude

Attitude is everything in recovery from cancer. You gotta have 'tude if you expect to take a licking and come back ticking.

Tumor humor is not warm and friendly; it's scrappy and sometimes nasty and tasteless, a sort of chemotherapy for the spirit—necessary but (not always) nice.

Robert Lipsyte

Reaching for the Best

Each human being possesses a beautiful system for fighting disease. This system provides the body with cancer-fighting cells—cells that can crush cancer cells or poison them one by one with the body's own chemotherapy. This system works better when the patient is relatively free of depression, which is what a strong will to live and a blazing determination can help to do. When we add these inner resources to the resources of medical science, we're reaching out for the best.

Norman Cousins

The Centerfold

My wife, Ellen, was lying in a hospital bed, a copy of *Playgirl* by her side. Suddenly, she opened to the male nude centerfold and insisted I put it on the wall.

"I think it's too risqué for the hospital, " I said.

"Nonsense," she replied. "Just take a leaf from the plant over there and cover up the genitals."

I did as she requested. This worked well for the first day. Everything was okay for the second day. By the third day, however, the leaf started to shrivel up and reveal more and more of what we were trying to conceal.

We laughed every time we looked at a plant or a dried-up leaf. The duration of our levity may have lasted only 10 or 20 seconds, but it brought us closer together, revived us and steered us through our sea of darkness.

Humor instantly took us away, even if only for moments, from our troubles and made them easier to bear. It gave us a breather. It was like a mini-vacation that allowed us to regain our strength and pull our resources together. Ellen's long illness was hardly a fun time; there were many tense and tearful moments, but there were also periods of laughter. Frequently she poked me in the ribs and admonished, "Hey, stop being so morose. I'm still here. We can still laugh together."

Allen Klein
from The Healing Power of Humor

The Power of Laughter

Ten minutes of genuine belly laughter had an anesthetic effect and would give me at least two hours of pain-free sleep.

Norman Cousins

Allison Crane, executive director of the American Association for Therapeutic Humor, recounts one story originally told to her by a middle-aged pastor:

> *I had a very serious accident a few years ago; it was amazing I survived. And, of course, I was in the hospital for a very long time recuperating.*
>
> *Because I was there for so long, I became rather nonchalant with the nurses about the procedures they subjected me to—you can't keep decorum up for very long with no clothes on. I was also having trouble finding a relatively painless spot to put yet another injection of pain medication. . . .*
>
> *One time I rang for the nurse, and when she came on the intercom, I told her I needed another pain shot. I knew it would take just about as long for her to draw up*

the medication as it would for me to gather the strength to roll over and find a spot for her to inject it. I had successfully rolled over, facing away from the door, when I heard her come in. "I think this area here isn't too bad," I said, pointing to an exposed area of my rear. But there was an awful silence after I said that. My face paled as I rolled over slowly to see who had actually come in— it was one of my 22-year-old female parishioners! I apologized and tried to chat with her, but she left shortly thereafter, horribly embarrassed.

Well, about 30 seconds after she left, the impact of the situation hit me and I started laughing. It hurt like you can't imagine, but I laughed and laughed and laughed. Tears rolled down my face and I was gasping when my nurse finally came in. She asked what had happened. I tried to tell her, but couldn't say more than a word or two before convulsing into laughing fits again. Amused, she told me she would give me a few minutes to calm down and she'd be back to give me my shot.

I had just regained my composure when my nurse reappeared and asked again what had happened. I started telling her, got to laughing again, and she started to laugh from just watching me, which made it worse. Finally, she left again, promising to try back in 15 more minutes. This scenario repeated itself a couple more times, and by the time I told her what had happened, I felt absolutely no pain. None. I didn't need medication for three more hours. And I know it was an emotional turning point in my recovery.

Allen Klein
from The Healing Power of Humor

Victim or Survivor

Although the definition said, "A cancer survivor is anyone who has ever been diagnosed with cancer and is alive today," the first time I read it, I didn't feel like a cancer survivor. Cancer victim seemed a much more accurate term. But then the dust settled, treatment began, and I realized the "victim" thing just didn't fit.

I tossed the victim/survivor issue around and finally came to the conclusion that a victim and a survivor are the same thing—almost. The differences are subtle but at the same time enormous. The first thing I realized is that a survivor is a victim with an attitude. After I understood that, things were a little better. I had a choice about something—I could be a cancer victim or a cancer survivor. I liked the idea of having an attitude and I liked the sound of being a survivor.

Next, I thought about a friend of mine who had metastatic breast cancer and was the epitome of a cancer survivor. To Barbie, survivorship was a state of mind. Despite the moments of sadness and pain, she never lost her ability to laugh about some of the absurdities of cancer and cancer treatment. She treasured every moment and faced each new situation as best as she could. Eventually, the cancer got her body; however, she never allowed it to reach her spirit. I think of her as a survivor in the truest sense of the word.

Very slowly, the differences between being a survivor and victim became clear, and I started making a list. I'm sure every survivor can add one or two more. This is just a start.

- Being a victim is a state of body. Being a survivor is a state of mind.
- A victim fears hair falling out. A survivor knows bald is beautiful.
- A victim knows about feeling down. A survivor knows feeling down is okay.
- A victim dreads the side effects of treatments. A survivor wonders how to cancel his membership in the Side-Effect-of-the-Month Club.
- A victim is amazed at all the tears. A survivor never leaves home without Kleenex.
- A victim goes to "see" a doctor. A survivor "consults" with his or her physician.
- A victim gets caught in despair. A survivor prays a lot.
- A victim feels helpless. A survivor says "thanks" with dignity and grace.
- A victim enjoys a good laugh. A survivor loves one.
- From the moment we are diagnosed, we are victims. We must *choose* to be survivors.

Paula (Bachleda) Koskey

4

ON FAITH

I have found that four faiths are crucial to recovery from serious illness: faith in oneself, one's doctor, one's treatment, and one's spiritual faith.

Bernie S. Siegel, M.D.

Going for the Prize

It takes a lot to get my mind off golf. Like most members of the Professional Golfers' Association, I eat, sleep and drink the game. That's the life of a pro. Or at least that's what I used to think.

Dr. Jobe called me unexpectedly on Friday evening after the second round of the 1993 PGA Championship at Inverness Club outside Toledo, Ohio. The PGA is a big tournament, one of the four "majors" (along with the Masters and the U.S. and British Opens).

At the time, I had the dubious distinction of being known as the best player in the world never to win a major. Sure, I had come a long way from salad days struggling to make the qualifying cut at the PGA "tour school." Back at the 1987 British Open, I had held the lead all week on the misty, windswept fairways of Muirfield in Scotland, only to suffer a devastating loss to Nick Faldo on the last hole. Though I won a lot of other tournaments, a major title still eluded me.

At age 33, I was at the top of my game and feeling pretty invincible. I was in good shape going into the third round at Inverness, just a couple of shots off the pace behind Greg "the Shark" Norman, an Australian. My family was in Ohio with me, which made golfing even more of a pleasure. It was a heady feeling competing for a $300,000 purse in front of a global TV audience. The pressure was definitely on. That's why it was strange that Dr. Jobe would call me at my hotel. My wife, Toni, handed me the receiver with a quizzical look and hushed the kids.

I had been having trouble again with nagging pain in my right shoulder. Dr. Jobe, one of the premier sports physicians in the world, had operated on my shoulder in 1991, and I had recently seen him in Los Angeles about the recurring soreness. Now he got right to the point: the X rays he had taken concerned him. "Paul, I want you back in Los Angeles for a biopsy as soon as possible." *Biopsy?* I thought. *Is he crazy? I'm in contention here. I have the rest of the tour to finish and the Ryder Cup. I can't take time off now!*

Dr. Jobe finally relented and agreed that the biopsy could wait until later in the fall, when I would be in California for a tournament. Until then I would survive on anti-inflammatories, aspirin and prayer. *Tendinitis,* I told myself, and banished it from my mind.

I went out the next day, a boiling hot Saturday, and shot a solid 68 to climb one stroke behind Norman. At the end of Sunday's final 18 holes, I was in a tie with the Shark for the Wanamaker Trophy. Then, on the second hole of sudden-death play, Greg missed a tricky putt for par and I made mine to become the PGA champ. I had my title! Not one to take things mildly, I leapt into the air. Next I gave thanks to the Lord, which is what I had always promised to do when I won a major. With Toni and our daughters, Sarah Jean, seven, and Josie, four, at my side, I went to raise the regal trophy high for all to see. Suddenly a sharp pain sliced through my right shoulder. It was all I could do to lift the silver cup.

I was determined not to let the pain lessen the thrill of victory or undermine my plans. I went to England and played with the United States team against the Europeans for the 1993 Ryder Cup, which we retained that year. But the pain never went away. By late November, when I finally saw Dr. Jobe in Los Angeles, I was barely able to operate the stick shift in my car. In fact, sometimes I drove and depressed the clutch while Toni shifted gears. As I sat on the table in Dr. Jobe's examining room that Monday morning at Centinela Hospital, showing him the spot on my shoulder that was now red-hot to the touch, he was irritated that he let me talk him out of doing a biopsy earlier. He took a pen and gently drew a line across the hot spot. "I'm going to make the incision right here," he said thoughtfully. "Don't shower that line off tomorrow morning."

As I dressed, for the first time I felt a stab of fear. *Come on, Zinger,* I reproached myself. *It's probably nothing.* That's what I told Toni that night back at the hotel while we talked quietly in our room and the kids went to dinner with Mildred, their sitter. What was the worst it could be? A stress fracture or some infection? I would be back on the course in no time. The next morning Dr. Jobe scraped out about a capful of tissue and bone for testing. We waited a few days for the results.

That week—a week of worry and prayer for Toni and me—I thought a lot about our life together and how intertwined with golf it was. We married in our home state of Florida in January of 1982 as soon as I got my tour card, and Toni was a golf wife from the start. In those hard, early years Toni and I traveled the country in an old camper, chasing the tournaments. In the off-season back in Florida, she worked as a bookkeeper while I practiced, practiced, practiced. It might be my name up there on the leader board when I'm playing well, but really, Toni's should be there too. She's been as much a part of my success as I have.

When Toni and I went back to see Dr. Jobe, I dispensed with the usual pleasantries. "How am I?" I blurted out.

He looked me right in the eye. "Paul, you have cancer."

One simple word. Cancer. Impossible. It was a good thing I was sitting. Toni gripped my hand and I rocked back and forth in my chair, shaking my head. I had been worried about my career, not about dying. Suddenly everything changed. "Paul, if the cancer is still localized, then it is treatable."

Something like a silent explosion overwhelmed me. "I need the restroom," I gasped, rushing out the door and down the hall. Bent over in that tiny bathroom, I put my head in my hands. I thought about Toni and the girls, about our life. I thought about golf. *Dear Lord, help me. I'm scared to death!* Then I cried until I heard Toni knocking on the door, asking gently, "Paul, are you okay?"

After I pulled myself together, Dr. Jobe brought me in to see an oncologist, Dr. Lorne Feldman, who put me through a battery of tests to determine if the cancer had spread beyond my shoulder. Late in the day, Toni and I went back to our hotel to struggle through a weekend of waiting for the test results. As I played with the kids I thought about the PGA title, and what a cruel twist it would be if it turned out that I should have been in the hospital instead of competing with Greg Norman in the heat and humidity at Inverness.

We took Sarah Jean and Josie to a mall on Saturday to take our minds off our situation, but all the Christmas decorations going up just made me more anxious. Early Sunday morning a false fire alarm roused us from bed. Toni noticed a sign in the lobby announcing church services in one of the ballrooms. "Want to go?" she asked me.

Toni and I had become Christians back in the days
when we were bouncing around the country in our old
camper—happy, carefree, uncomplicated days, they
seemed now. Sometimes it is when you have the least
that you are most aware of how much the Lord provides.
We always managed to put enough food in our mouths
and gas in the camper. We took turns driving and reading
aloud from the Bible.

Now Toni, Mildred, the kids and I slipped quietly into
the back of the ballroom where services were being held
by a local church whose regular facilities were under con-
struction. The big room was full and smelled of cut flowers. That false alarm had not been so false after all. There
was a fire in the air, a spiritual charge I felt throughout
my body. I sensed I was face to face with God, and an
excitement I hadn't felt in years came over me. I knew
that Christ wanted not just my cancer, or my golf, or my
fears about my family, but all of it—my whole life, if only
I would give it to him and recommit myself to faith. *I need
you now more than ever, Lord,* I whispered silently.

That afternoon my parents flew in from Florida, and the
next day we got the news from Dr. Feldman that as far as
they could determine the cancer had not spread beyond
the right scapula. I was immediately scheduled for six
chemotherapy treatments, one every four weeks, admin-
istered right there in his office, starting that day. Between
treatments I could return home to Florida.

That first chemo session was a doozy. I suffered
intractable nausea and got so dehydrated that I had to be
rushed back to the hospital for emergency treatment. But
after a few days, Toni and I flew home. Coming home is
always a relief to a professional athlete, the real reward at
the end of the game. This time it was even more so.

Anyone who has seen me golf knows I am not a player
who disguises his emotions. You don't need the TV

commentator to tell you if I am happy or upset with a shot. I'll let you know. That's me, not exactly Mr. Mellow. Yet the first few days home, I found myself spending hours in our backyard just looking at the flowers and the trees, or watching birds through binoculars. I was getting so mellow it was beginning to scare me! "Maybe the chemo went to my brain," I told Toni, joking.

The phone rang regularly with well-wishers, including President Bush and even my PGA competitor Greg Norman. I found out that the Shark has a soft side.

Then one morning while I was getting ready for the day, something happened. I stood in my bedroom praying, wondering in the back of my mind what would happen if I didn't get better. The sun was forcing its way through the blinds when suddenly, a powerful feeling swelled over me like a huge, gently rolling wave lifting my feet off the sand bottom of the sea. I stopped everything I was doing and experienced an incredible, peace-giving sensation. I knew that God was with me, and I felt absolutely assured that I would be okay. It wasn't that God told me what would happen next or that the cancer would go away. I simply felt positive I was in his complete and loving care no matter what.

I am blessed to say that today, two years after my diagnosis, the cancer is gone. I'm back on the tour trying to shake the rust off my golf game. Dr. Jobe said it was probably a good thing I didn't rush out to California right after the PGA title because at that time, the number of cancer cells in my body might not have been sufficient to show up on a biopsy. I guess in a way, my competitive drive saved me after all, but what keeps me going most these days is the chance to be an example for others who are struck by disease, to help them see that God is there for them no matter what. That's all you need to know to get through anything in life. That is the real "major."

Which is not to say, of course, that the next time I find myself in a playoff with the Shark you won't be able to tell how I feel about a shot. I am the way God made me, and I don't think the Lord is interested in tinkering with my golf game.

Paul Azinger

Say a Prayer

I was taking my usual morning walk when a garbage truck pulled up beside me. I thought the driver was going to ask for directions. Instead, he showed me a picture of a cute little five-year-old boy. "This is my grandson, Jeremiah," he said. "He's on a life-support system at a Phoenix hospital." Thinking he would next ask for a contribution to his hospital bills, I reached for my wallet. But he wanted something more than money. He said, "I'm asking everybody I can to say a prayer for him. Would you say one for him, please?" I did. And my problems didn't seem like much that day.

Bob Westenberg

On Faith

Pray to God, but row for shore.

Russian proverb

Phyllis, a patient who had an extensive pancreatic cancer that was no longer responding to treatment, went home to die. Several months later she returned to the office. One of my partners examined her. He opened the door of the examining room and called me: "Hey, Bernie, you're interested in this stuff."

I came in and he said, "Her cancer's gone."

"Phyllis," I said, "tell them what happened."

She said, "Oh, you know what happened."

"I know that I know," I said, "but I'd like the others to know."

Phyllis replied, "I decided to live to be a hundred and leave my troubles to God."

Peace of mind can heal anything. I believe faith is the essence, a simple solution, yet too hard for most people to practice.

To verify this I went to God (surgeons have that prerogative) and asked why I couldn't hang a sign in my waiting room saying, "Leave your troubles to God, you don't need me." God said, "I'll show you why. I'll meet you at the hospital at 10 A.M. Saturday." (God likes to play doctor.)

On Saturday he said, "Take me to your sickest patient." I told him about a woman with cancer whose husband had run off with another woman. He said, "Good case," and we went up to her room.

I said, "Ma'am, God is going to come in and tell you how to get well. I always introduce him so patients are not overwhelmed."

She responded, "Oh, wonderful."

God entered the room and said, "All you have to do is love, accept, forgive and choose to be happy."

She looked him in the eye and said, "Have you met my husband yet?"

Most of us want God to change the external aspects of our lives so that we don't have to change internally. We want to be exempt from the responsibility for our own happiness. We often find it easier to resent and suffer in the role of victim than to love, forgive, accept and find inner peace. As W. H. Auden has written,

We would rather be ruined than changed;
We would rather die in our dread
Than climb the cross of the moment
And let our illusions die.

Yet, when we choose to love, healing energy is released in our bodies. Energy itself is loving and intelligent and available to all of us.

Now I felt I had a dilemma: If God's love could cure people, I wondered, why should I remain a surgeon? So I returned to him and said, "God, you know one of my patients got well leaving her troubles to you. Why should I remain a surgeon? Why not just teach people to love?"

And God in his beautiful sweet, melodious voice said to me, "Bernie, render unto the surgeon what is the surgeon's, and render unto God what is God's." (I find that God does that a lot—speaks in parables and leaves you totally confused.) Since then I've come to understand that God and I both have a role in getting people well.

Let me illustrate what I mean with an old story I've adapted.

A man with cancer is told by his primary physician he'll be dead in an hour. He runs to the window, looks up at the sky, and says, "God, save me." Out of the blue comes that wonderful melodious voice saying, "Don't worry, my son. I will save you." The man climbs back into bed, feeling reassured.

His physician calls me and I walk in and say, "If I operate in an hour, I can save you."

"No thanks," says the man, "God will save me."

Then the oncologist, a radiation therapist and a nutritional therapist all tell him, "We can save you."

"I don't need you, God will save me," is his reply to all of them.

In an hour the man dies. When he gets to heaven, he walks up to God and says, "What happened? You said you'd save me, and here I am dead."

"You dumbbell. I did try to save you. I sent you a surgeon, an oncologist, a radiation therapist and a nutritional therapist."

Bernie S. Siegel, M.D.

The Holy Water

Lola was a humor therapist at the time of her diagnosis, so she said her immediate reaction was to find the humor where possible and encourage her friends to do the same. One instance stayed with her.

"I'm Catholic, but go to church anonymously because I don't want to get involved. I just like to go. Someone gave me some holy water from Lourdes back before the cancer, and I was in the habit of blessing my husband before he left for work. For fun, you know—'Wait, you haven't been blessed.' Well, I ran out of water and wanted some and didn't want to ask the priest. So I took my little bottle and filled it from the font after everyone left the church. I told my friend I felt bad about stealing holy water. Anyway, after my biopsy she said it was because I got hold of some bad holy water, and when I woke up after surgery there was a big poinsettia from her and a juice jug of holy water. I still have some in my closet. It's got algae growing on the bottom, but I can't bear to get rid of it."

Kathy LaTour

Great Expectations

Faith is to believe what we do not see; the reward of this faith is to see what we believe.

Saint Augustine

May 1st was supposed to be a day of happy excitement, the day I would bring my husband home to our little town in Arkansas from the big city hospital in Memphis. Instead, the doctor had unexpectedly scheduled Byzie for his fourth surgery in six months. Byzie came through it all right. But the uncertainty of his situation—an unfinished battle with cancer—kept me from feeling any relief. Now I sat in the intensive care waiting room. In two hours, I could spend 15 minutes with him.

My thoughts turned to our children many miles away, making do at home while I stayed with Byzie. I found myself remembering a bleak conversation with the two oldest girls after they'd heard the news of their father's latest surgery.

"When one member of a family has cancer, it's as if the whole family has it," 16-year-old Kathey had said forlornly.

Karen, our 17-year-old, nodded sadly. "Now Dad won't make it home in time for my graduation, will he?"

Karen was right. It was unlikely that Byzie would be home by May 10. And Kathey was right about the contagious effect of Byzie's illness. Our four children, taking their cue from me, became more despondent each day. Kristen, six, clinged too tightly, cried too easily. Alan, nine, had nightmares.

I fumbled for a tissue and forced myself to look about the waiting room. A surgeon in green operating room coveralls strode in and began talking in muted tones to the string of family members that quickly knotted around him. One of them was obviously the mother: tall, finely chiseled, with silver hair. She swayed against one of the two young men on either side of her, then straightened and began walking unassisted toward an empty cluster of chairs near me. Her family followed.

I grabbed an outdated magazine and shrank back into my chair. I would not intrude on their sorrow; I did not want them to trespass on mine.

Hidden behind my magazine, I let the painful memories come back. First Byzie had tests; then came the diagnosis, and one of the ugliest words in Webster's entered our lives.

Through the early stages, faith and assurance were strong. The major word in our household was *when: when* Dad would go fishing with Alan, *when* Dad would fix Kristen's bike. I tried remembering the exact moment that *when* had become *if.* Summer . . . autumn and icy winter had disappeared. Now pink and white dogwood blossoms trembled on their branches. A neighbor had fixed Kristen's bike; friends took Alan fishing. *If* was changing to *never* in my mind.

My magazine slipped to the floor and I buried my face in my hands, forgetting the family next to me. *Father,* I prayed silently, *I don't want to be like Job's wife, but everything seems so hopeless. Please help me.*

A clean linen handkerchief was pressed into my hand. "Here, honey, some cries take more than a tissue."

Startled, then embarrassed, I couldn't stop sobbing. The handkerchief was as wilted as I was when I finally looked up into a sea of black faces and concerned brown-velvet eyes. Six young adults—three women and three men—and their mother had positioned their chairs in a semicircle around me. One of the men handed me a steaming cup of coffee. Introductions were made. They were the Turner family.

"I'm sorry," I said. "I lost control for a moment. I'll be all right."

"I know you will." Mrs. Turner smiled sympathetically. "Sounds like you're to the point of having to get by on evidence now."

I must have looked confused.

"She doesn't know what you mean, Mama," one of the daughters said, "Not many people know Papa's way of believing."

A ripple of laughter ran through their midst. As they explained, I was drawn into their family circle.

John, the Turners' father, had been reared on a dusty cotton plantation in Mississippi. He wanted to leave and go to the city, but it all seemed hopeless until the night he attended a "shouting and singing brush-arbor revival meeting." The sweating evangelist had heated the ancient definition of faith to a red-hot pitch—"Now faith is the substance of things hoped for, the evidence of things not seen" (Hebrews 11:1)—and those words seared his heart and mind.

After John loped home that summer evening, he rummaged around and found an empty fruit jar. He placed it by his bed. This would be the "evidence" of his faith. Little by little he would place money in that jar. God would help him fill it as many times as it took to start his journey to a new opportunity. And so, dozens of odd jobs and acres of farm work later, the jar was filled enough times for him to move to the city, to find a job with the railroad, to meet and marry the woman who was talking to me now.

"He bought a picture frame with a cardboard backing and hung it on our apartment wall, over the crack in the plaster. He said the deed for our home would hang in it someday." Mrs. Turner's voice broke. A daughter picked up the story.

"And after each of us was born, he hung up two empty frames—one for our high school and one for our college diploma." She chuckled. "We're probably the only family in the world that decorated our walls with empty frames. We had 13 of them as 'evidence of things not seen.'"

Now the oldest-looking son spoke up. "But Papa kept saying that during hard times, when your spirits might slip, that's when you needed to look at some evidence that proved your faith hadn't."

Nine frames had been filled so far, the young man said, "and Annie and Kate are in college and Terrence is a senior in high school."

Mrs. Turner's voice was as soft as her expression. "I'm no Bible scholar but my husband is right. God doesn't always send signs; sometimes you have to put them up yourself. He sees them and knows that you believe, even when you can't see around the curve in the road. And He honors that. A lot of John's signs are visible, but a lot more are in here." She pointed to her heart.

A buzzer sounded. Visiting time had arrived. Mrs. Turner and I walked to the receptionist's desk to collect our passes. I began walking away, then turned and looked at Mrs. Turner. I couldn't speak.

She opened her arms and I clung to her strength—for

just a moment. Then I hurried down the hall to Byzie's room. Tubes dangled from his chest and other parts of his body. His eyes were closed. I sat down carefully at his bedside.

In the waiting silence, I thought of Noah standing in swirling dust, pounding away on a gopher-wood ark. And Abraham piling up giant altar stones in a strange new land. And John Turner filling an empty fruit jar and hanging empty frames.

Currents of excitement tingled through me. All of these men displayed visible evidence of an invisible faith force. This same force was inside the very core of my life, right where the "substance of things hoped for" was stored. A force that nothing—nothing—could destroy.

Byzie's eyes opened. "Are you okay?" he asked. I could tell it hurt him to talk.

"Honey, I'm more okay than I've been in ages."

Byzie smiled and shut his eyes again. The 15 minutes were up; I tiptoed away.

After leaving intensive care, I rushed to a pay phone and called long distance to our home. Karen answered. "Tell Alan and Kristen to paint a 'Welcome Home' sign," I burst out. "And have Kathey buy some big balloons and crêpe paper streamers. I don't know when, but your dad is coming home!"

"Oh, Mom," Karen said, her voice choking. "I was almost afraid to get my hopes up."

"I was too," I admitted. "But I'll never be afraid to hope again." I promised to write a long letter that evening, explaining my change of heart.

I hung up the phone and went to the hospital gift shop where, by good luck, I found what I was looking for—a small ceramic figure of a girl graduate with "Class of 81" embossed at the base. On my next visit to Byzie that evening, I placed it on the window ledge.

On May 10th Byzie sat at my side in the auditorium. He wore a snowy carnation, a gift from Karen, in his lapel. As the strains of "Pomp and Circumstance" rang out, we watched our daughter enter, smiling more brightly than any of us.

I knew we had rough days ahead, but I also knew that my faith would always be more contagious than any disease that could strike our family. I would keep it in my heart and I would display it by my actions. Evidence for God—and everyone—to see.

Jeanette Doyle Parr

I Said a Prayer for You Today

I said a prayer for you today
    And know God must have heard—
I felt the answer in my heart
    Although He spoke no word!
I didn't ask for wealth or fame
    (I knew you wouldn't mind)—
I asked Him to send treasures
    Of a far more lasting kind!
I asked that He'd be near you
    At the start of each new day
To grant you health and blessings
    And friends to share your way!
I asked for happiness for you
    In all things great and small—
But it was for His loving care
    I prayed the most of all!

Source Unknown

Don't Worry—Be Happy

Why is it when we talk to God we are said to be praying, and when God talks to us we're said to be schizophrenic?

Lily Tomlin

In December 1991, I was diagnosed with rectal cancer, which had grown from its earlier stages because of my initial reluctance to have it examined by a doctor. By mid-January 1992 I was operated on for a colon re-section.

During the spring and summer I concentrated on healing, but things inside just weren't right and I knew it. I experienced pain and too many bowel movements each day. A medical procedure searched for the cause, and another procedure opened my rectum. The doctors decided a colostomy was in order. By this time I was pretty tired of being a hospital "bird," and wanted to get it all over with and get on with my life. A third operation was scheduled.

By March 1993, I had my new colostomy and also some bad news. During my operation, the doctor saw cancerous looking tissue but couldn't deal with it and do my colostomy too, so he took some biopsies and closed me up. The biopsies revealed the cancer had returned to the same place (the rectal area) and was spreading. I was depressed beyond belief. It was a rainy, dreary March morning and I watched the feeble light of dawn from my rain-streaked windows. I was depressed and in despair. Lying in the hospital, my doctor's words rang in my ears. "It's a can of worms down there, Paul—you'll need another operation by a skilled team of surgeons who just do this kind of pelvic surgery. I can't do it."

I had always shunned religion and was forever trying to prove a Godless universe to anyone who took the positive view. I was an empiricist and was proud of my intellectual detachment. But lying there that morning full of hopelessness and sick of it all, I asked for God's help.

In a moment, I drifted back into that twilight sleep and I was suddenly surprised to find myself standing on a downtown street complete with sidewalks and curbs. "This is no dream," I thought. "I am really here on this typical American street corner looking around." Just then three people appeared from across the street, walking my way. It was two men and a woman. As they got closer to me, the men sat down on the curb and began talking with each other. The woman came right up to me, smiling and giving out such a force of joy and love that I was completely taken by her presence. She put her arm around me and I felt heavenly bliss. An intense concern and love emanated from her body, completely enthralling me. She was beautiful. Her eyes were brown and her dark hair was cut short, reminding me of Prince Valiant. With her arm around me she looked into my eyes and said, "You're going to be all right now, no more medical problems. Be happy, don't worry. Everything's going to be okay. Please be happy and don't worry." Then, as we stood there, it was clear that my time was over and they were going to leave. The two men stood up and all three began walking away. I remember how earnestly I implored them to stay. The woman was the last to leave and she turned to me again and said, "Don't worry, be happy. Everything's going to be all right."

Eight months and a series of chemo treatments later, a team of three surgeons at a medical center in Portland, Oregon opened me up (my fourth operation) and found not a trace of cancer—even though only months before both CAT scans and MRI's had found the cancer reaching for my prostate, my bladder and the whole pelvic area. All three doctors were extremely surprised and delighted by what they didn't find. I was absolutely clean—the biopsies that were taken then all came back negative.

Paul Santaro

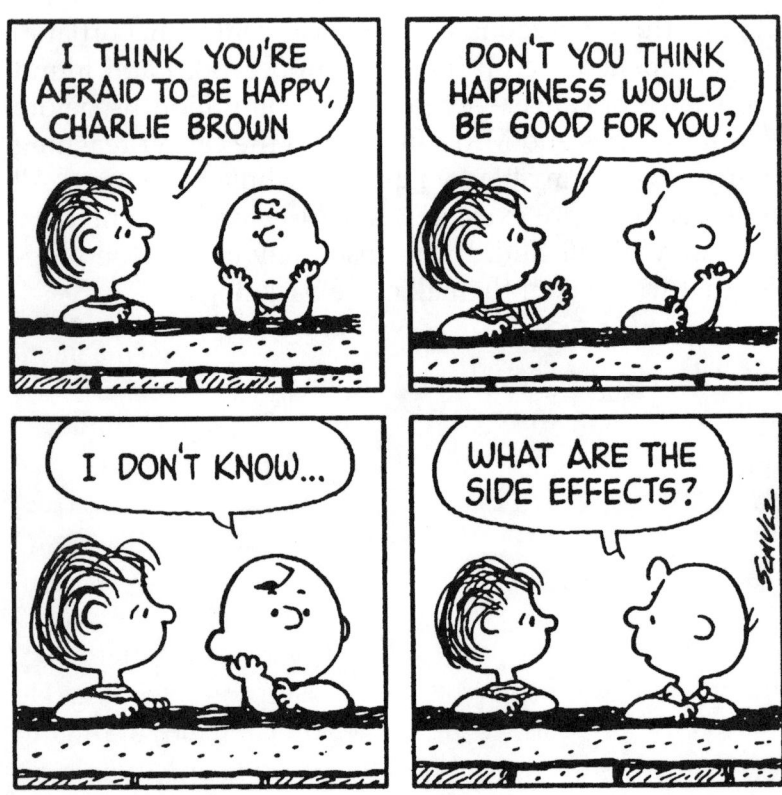

All the Necessary Supplies

Very early on Sunday morning, March 29, 1992, I was up again with our nine-year-old son, Nicholas. I spent a couple hours trying to stop yet another bloody nose. We had been going through this routine now for about six weeks. Doctors had diagnosed the trouble as a sinus infection, which we had been treating since February. Just the Friday before, we had been to the doctor's office again.

By 7:30 A.M. that Sunday, my husband and I decided to drive Nicholas to the hospital emergency room about 25 miles from our home. With some difficulty, the emergency room doctor cauterized the area to stop the bleeding. He was ready to send us home when I felt an urging to request a blood test. Nicholas had been losing quite a bit of blood and was so tired and listless I thought he might be anemic. After the blood was drawn, we were told we could go home, and the lab would notify us if anything showed up. We decided we would just wait for the results.

The waiting was much longer than we anticipated. Finally, the emergency room doctor came in and said he was calling in the pediatrician on call because something had shown up in the blood work. Immediately I knew it must be leukemia, but didn't say anything to my husband. Soon the pediatrician came in and confirmed my fears. In a state of shock we drove home, packed some clothes, made a few phone calls to family and friends, and were on our way to Primary Children's Medical Center in Salt Lake City, Utah. Though it is about a four-and-a-half hour trip from our southern Idaho home, that trip seemed to last days.

Nicholas was diagnosed with acute lymphoblastic leukemia and spent four days in intensive care and two more days on the floor. He received wonderful care and the doctors assured us that the odds were in his favor, even though they initially thought he had a poor prognosis. They outlined the three-year treatment consisting of brain radiation and chemotherapy.

At home again, I tried to get back into some kind of routine and semblance of normalcy. I turned the page of a meditation calendar a dear friend had given me for Christmas. It was open to March 29, the day Nicholas was diagnosed. The message for that day: "All the necessary supplies have already been planned and provided for this journey." I found great comfort and reassurance. I felt God had provided this message.

It has been over three years now and Nicholas just finished treatment. There have been many ups and downs along the way and many wonderful acts of kindness. Always I come back to that message—"All the necessary supplies have already been planned and provided for this journey." And they have been!

Dianne Clark

5

ON LOVE

There is no difficulty that enough love will not conquer; no disease that enough love will not heal; no door that enough love will not open; no gulf that enough love will not bridge; no wall that enough love will not throw down; no sin that enough love will not redeem. . . .

It makes no difference how deeply seated may be the trouble; how hopeless the outlook; how muddled the tangle; how great the mistake. A sufficient realization of love will dissolve it all. If only you could love enough you would be the happiest and most powerful being in the world.

Emmet Fox

Eileen Brown's Story

I can still remember the day I found out. I called my doctor. It was 4:15 on a Thursday afternoon. I had just finished my last bite of a Hostess cupcake when the receptionist answered the phone. "Doctor's office, can I help you?"

"Yes, this is Eileen Brown. I'm calling for the results of my tests."

"Hold on a minute. The doctor is with a patient."

"Wait a minute," I said, as I was put on hold, "I don't have to talk to the doctor. You can give me my results." *I'm going to be late for class and I'll never find a place to park,* I thought. *I don't see why the nurse can't say everything's negative. After all, I took the mammography last week. If anything was wrong, the doctor would have called me by now.*

"Hi, Eileen."

"Hi, Doc, so what's the good word? I'm in a hurry to get to school, so tell me everything is fine, and I can get going."

"Not so fast, Eileen. I've been trying to reach you for three days. There's a growth on your right breast." I felt the bottom of my stomach drop out. In shock, all I could think was, *Oh, please God, don't let me need an operation. I'm so terrified of being put to sleep. What if I slip into a coma?*

"Eileen, did you hear me?" the doctor's voice brought me back to earth.

"Yes, but it's nothing, right? I don't need an operation, right?" I said.

"Eileen, the lump has to come out."

I heard myself begging. "Please, you're not telling me cancer, are you?" *Please, God, not my breast, I can't lose my breast.*

"I'm not pulling any punches with you, Eileen. From the looks of the X rays and the written report, there is a malignancy at 12 o'clock on your right breast. I've scheduled an appointment for Saturday morning with Dr. Johnson*, a breast surgeon at NYU."

Numb, I hung up the phone, ran downstairs to the basement, sat on the cold cement floor and cried. I felt as if I was having an out-of-body experience. I must be watching someone else. This could not be happening to me, not now. My husband, Bob, and I were still newlyweds (only married for 16 months). I had three beautiful children from my first marriage, a family I loved very much, and a great new job teaching. I clutched my breast through my tear-stained blouse. *I don't want to leave my family, not now. I'm not ready to die,* I thought.

In the days that followed, my family and close friends tried to convince themselves and me that the growth was nothing and the doctors were wrong. Thoughts of death raced through our minds, but we were all too afraid to verbalize them. The week was a total blur as we went about our lives and waited for the appointment with Dr. Johnson. When the day finally arrived, my family accompanied me to his office. Dr. Johnson confirmed the report and told us he would perform an aspiration, a procedure in which a needle is inserted into the breast and fluid and

---

* Dr. Johnson's name has been changed to protect his identity.

tissue are taken from the lump.

The 20 minutes it would take to get the results back seemed like an eternity. I paced the floor of the cafeteria where we went to spend the time.

"Eileen, sit down and have a cold drink. All we can do now is wait," said my father.

"I don't have to wait to be told I have cancer. We all know that now. What we're waiting for is a tiny thread of hope. I can't drink or put anything in my mouth. I just want to run away, but . . . I guess I can't run from myself," I said.

After about 25 minutes of sheer agony, we went back to Dr. Johnson's office. I wasn't prepared for the reception I got there. "Where were you?" he asked, brusquely. "You know, some people would like to get out of here and go home."

"What are the results, doctor?" I asked, shocked.

"It's malignant and I'm removing your breast a week from today." Bob's hand went to my shoulder and the tears began to fall.

I said, "Doctor, do you think maybe you could give me something to calm me down until the surgery?"

Coldly, he said, "Sorry, I don't believe in taking pills to mask your feelings. You're going to have to learn to get along without it anyway, and you may as well start now."

The four of us left the hospital in silence. Bob held my hand as my mother and father wept. We drove to my mother's house in Brooklyn where my brothers and sister were waiting for the outcome.

My sister, Karen, took the news worst of all. Everyone cried but had accepted the fact. She was unable to. "They made a mistake," she said, running away from me. I followed her from room to room, grabbed her by the shoulders and said, "Every doctor didn't make a mistake and every test is not wrong. You've been running away from this for a week and it's time you stopped running. I have cancer!" With this, her legs buckled and she started sobbing uncontrollably as I held her and tried to comfort her. I always considered myself a weak person, unable to deal with any kind of crisis. I was certainly not the one to give strength to others. It was at this point, however, that I realized I had to be strong because everyone was looking to me for their cues. As long as I didn't let myself cry, they would be afraid to cry in front of me. We learned to use the nights and our times alone to cry. In the daylight, and for each other, we would all be strong.

Bob and I went home. I told the kids—Scott, 16; Adam, 14; and Corinne, 7—that I needed an operation but would be fine. How do you discuss removing a breast with your sons and daughter?

That night I felt an overwhelming need to get my affairs in order so I straightened out my closet. I didn't want anyone else to have to clean up my life. All those special cards, pressed flowers and mementos that would mean nothing to anyone but me were put into the garbage. When it was time for bed, Bob held me as I lay silently weeping. I reached up to touch his face and realized that I wasn't the only person crying that night. Our fears were confirmed.

The night passed. The sun rose the next day as usual. The kids got ready for school. Bob and I dressed for work. Before I left the house, I got a call from Jeff, my ex-husband. He told me about an article in *Good Housekeeping* that listed the best breast cancer surgeons in the country. It included a female doctor, Alison Goldfarb, who was affiliated with Mt. Sinai Hospital near our home. After my experience with Dr. Johnson, Jeff suggested that maybe a woman would have more compassion in this type of surgery. Later that day, I called Dr. Goldfarb and made an appointment the next day for a second opinion.

My mother and sister went with me to Dr. Goldfarb's office and came after my examination into the consultation room. Dr. Goldfarb said she wanted me to have a reconstruction done immediately after the surgery, as I was still a young woman. My entire body shook. I cried tears of joy. She was the only doctor who held out any hope or spoke of the future to me—the only one who made me feel like I was going to live. I asked her to be my doctor.

Dr. Goldfarb smiled warmly and quickly got me an appointment with a reconstructive surgeon, Dr. Skolnik. He showed us slides of different breasts, all shapes and sizes. There were women who had reconstruction with and without nipples. We couldn't see the women's faces, only their disfigured breasts. "That doesn't look so bad, right?" I said, to my mother who was sitting behind me. I turned to her for confirmation. She looked horrified, an image that was a direct reflection of my own feelings. Being in the room together prevented us from falling apart. We tried hard to be brave for each other.

After hearing of the different options for reconstruction, I chose the procedure with the least amount of surgery. It involved placing a balloon under my skin and filling it with saline solution. The skin would stretch around the balloon and form a breast. The nipple would be added later. An appointment was set up for me to take pictures for the "before" shots. I was told to remove my necklace so I could not be identified. I, too, would be one of the faceless women in the slides.

My surgery was now two weeks away. I was torn between wanting the time to fly by and wanting it to stop where it was. There were so many things I needed to handle before then.

One of the details I had to take care of was telling Mr. Russo, the principal of the school where I worked, what was happening. I was very nervous about losing a full-time job that I had received just one month before. I had been a substitute in the school, working on a day-to-day basis, and was given the opportunity for a full-time job when one of the teachers had to take the rest of the year off. I promised the principal that I would be there every day without fail. Now I had to tell him that I had cancer and would need a month off.

Nervously, I approached Mr. Russo, choking back tears, and told him of my situation. His response touches me to this day. "Don't cry, there is nothing more important than your health," he said. "You take as long as you need. I'll get a substitute to cover your class. When you feel up to coming back, it will be waiting for you." I still can't believe he got a substitute to cover for a substitute.

I also needed to prepare for my hospital stay. My mother and sister took me shopping for nightgowns and a robe. They spared no expense. Anything that I wanted or felt good in was mine. Walking through the store, I overheard a woman commenting to her companion about the high price of a dress. "I'd only pay *that* price for a dress if I were dying of cancer," she said. "Then I wouldn't have to worry about getting the bill." My mother's face was sheet white.

I said, "Mom, I heard what they said. It's okay. They couldn't know."

After school on Friday, I had to go to the hospital for pre-op testing. There were blood tests, urine tests, a cardiogram and a chest X ray to be taken. Fear gripped me as I was called in to take the chest X ray. *What if it's in my lungs, too?* I thought. I started to shake so uncontrollably that blankets were put around me. I played a mind game with myself. If they didn't have to redo the X ray, then there was nothing wrong. But then, they didn't have to redo my mammography.

As my surgery grew closer, we all went through the motions and carried on with our daily routines as best we could. For me, showers were the hardest. Each day I was forced to wash and touch this thing that might be taking my life. I would stand frozen as the water mixed with my salty tears. When I was finally cried-out, I would stand in front of the mirror to dry myself and start over. It was part of me. When it was time to leave the bathroom, I had to paint on a smile and act as if nothing was wrong. I couldn't let my children know the fear I felt inside.

Bob bore the brunt of my feelings. He was my release, my savior. Bob was the one I snapped at and took my frustrations out on. He knew I was a walking time bomb ready to explode. I needed someone to tell my fears to.

On Monday morning, I received an urgent message: "Call Dr. Goldfarb immediately, very important." The room swayed, and I felt everything going black. Something was wrong with my tests. They found something else. I just knew it.

As it turned out, nothing was wrong with the tests. Due to a cancellation, Dr. Goldfarb had an opening in her surgical schedule the next morning at nine o'clock—a week ahead of my scheduled surgery.

"Trust me, Eileen, this is a blessing in disguise for you," said Dr. Goldfarb. "Next week at this time, it will all be behind you."

"I can't do it. I just can't. I don't have slippers. I'm not ready. Dear God, I'm not ready!"

"Eileen, you don't need slippers. You can have the surgery, then we'll get your slippers. Please listen to me and save yourself a lot of grief. I'll meet you at the hospital at 7:00." I agreed and then called Bob and my mother to let them know what was happening.

I drove home from school in a daze. I kept myself as busy as I could until Bob got home. I vacuumed, dusted, packed my overnight bag, washed and set my hair, shaved my legs and cried.

I didn't get many phone calls that night because everyone was afraid to talk to me. They didn't know what to say or how to say it. I told Adam and Corinne that I had to take more tests in the city and that Aunt Shelley would pick them up after school.

Through the night, Bob held me and reassured me that nothing would change for him as long as he still had me. He said he loved all of me, not just one part. He told me that I was beautiful on the inside as well as on the outside, and no operation could ever change that. No matter what Bob said, I still felt as though I was short-changing him. He deserved a whole woman, one with two breasts. We clung to each other that night, each of us getting and giving support at the same time. I knew that no matter what happened the next day, my family would be there for me. Their love was truly unconditional.

When the sun rose the next morning, Bob and I got dressed in silence. We were afraid to speak because the kids were getting ready for school. The ride to the hospital was tense and silent. We didn't know what to say. Bob was driving the speed limit, but it felt like we got there much too soon. I needed more time. I wasn't ready. Would I ever be ready?

We parked the car and went inside. My mother, father, sister and Aunt Florence were already there; they were afraid of missing me before I had to go upstairs. We all kissed and held each other. Nobody wanted to be the first to cry or let go. The only words spoken were "I love you."

I was taken into a room to change and put on a gown, and an I.V. was started. I sat on the bed and tried to make idle talk with my mother and aunt. I couldn't hear what was being said to me. The loud beating of my heart drowned out everything. I was allowed to wait with my family in the sitting room until an orderly was sent to get me.

At 8:45 a gurney arrived; it was time. We all kissed and clung to each other. *My God, they can open me up and find that the cancer has spread,* I thought. The doctor let Mom and

Bob go upstairs with me. I clung to their hands; they were my lifeline but I had to let go. I had been brave and strong up until this point, but now, in the upstairs pre-op area, I felt the weight of the last weeks. God, how I didn't want to let go of my mother's hand. She would take care of me. All that would come out of my lips was "I'm scared!" The tears began to fall and at that moment I knew the real meaning of fear. Mom and Bob both kissed me and told me how much they loved me. Bob put his arm around my mother to support her. It made me feel better to know they were there for each other.

We were only upstairs in the holding area for about five minutes when they were told they had to leave. I thought, *Please don't leave me here, I feel so alone. Oh, God, I'm on my own now. I can still get off the gurney and run. But where can I run to? My legs are paralyzed. My whole body is paralyzed with fear.* The lights blinded me as I was wheeled into the operating room.

Dr. Goldfarb came to my side and took my hand. "I'm right here with you, Eileen. I'm just moving around to the other side." I closed my eyes and thought, *Don't take the wrong one.*

God was good to me. I slept peacefully. My surgery was much longer than anticipated and lasted until five that evening, but it went very well. Eleven lymph nodes were removed and luckily the cancer had not metastasized.

The first person I saw after the operation was my sister, Karen. God, how her smile lit up the whole floor. She called to the rest of the family, "She's here. She's here. Hurry." As she ran to my side, Karen looked down at me and said, "You're beautiful. You look so beautiful." To this day, I have never or will never feel as beautiful as I did at that moment. I looked in her eyes and I knew that's how she saw me.

I got so many flowers and cards during my stay in the hospital that staff and patients thought I was someone famous or important. They were right. I was very important to a lot of people.

I had my mastectomy on Tuesday morning, left the hospital Saturday morning, and went right to the beauty parlor to have my hair done. After all, I had a birthday party to go to on Sunday. I started chemo two weeks after my operation, and I never missed a day of school during that time. It wasn't easy. I lost my hair. I threw up and felt sick. I had many times when I felt full of self-pity and said, "I can't do it anymore. I can't finish the chemo." I remember one day crying on the phone to my mother. "What happens if after going through all of this, it comes back?"

My mother replied, "Your children need you. You'll do whatever you have to do to be with them." She was right. Not only did my children need me—I needed them, too. They gave me the strength to fight and go on. I had a very good life and I wasn't ready to cash in my chips yet. I want to see my children go to college, get married and have families of their own. I want to grow old with my husband. I love my life and I intend to be here for a long time and make the most of each day.

Eileen Brown O'Riley

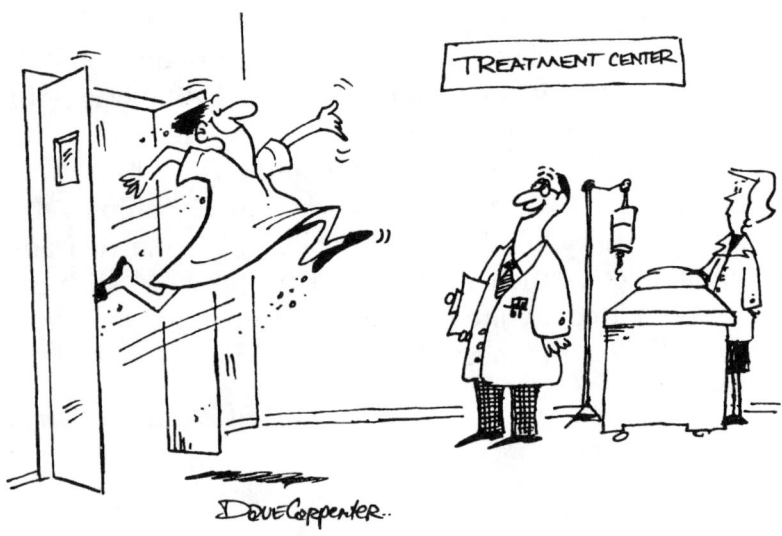

"I must admit, Mr. Feldmond, I like your attitude!"

A Pocket Full of Quarters

Searra, an eight-year-old brain tumor patient, was a "regular" in the Radiation Oncology Department, much like the other patients who came to the cancer center everyday for a five- or six-week period. With my office located near the main entrance, I could hear Searra, also called CC, coming from a distance.

Sure enough, she popped her head in every morning around 10:00 A.M. to say "hi" or, more important, to check out the toys and coloring materials I had stashed in my office. Several steps behind, CC's grandmother, also called Mommie, since she served as her guardian, would trail in as she tried keeping up with CC's anxious pace.

CC was not the least bit interested in hearing more about her cancer or her hair loss. When she walked into the department, it was time to socialize with the staff, who became her instant friends, and to see what kind of masterpiece she could color for Mommie before she was called back for her treatment.

I was taken aback by the love CC had for Mommie. Whenever I asked her about home life, school work or how she was feeling, every response referred to her time spent with Mommie, the funny stories they shared and how much she loved her. On numerous occasions, CC made it clear that Mommie was the center of her world.

When CC was first treated with radiation therapy, the therapists told her that they would give her a quarter each day if she promised to keep her head still on the treatment table. Certainly, after six weeks of therapy, she had a pocketful of quarters! So on the last day, the therapists wanted to know what big toy she was going to buy with all her change. CC replied, "Oh, I am not going to buy a toy. I am going to buy something for Mommie because of all the nice things she does for me."

CC's sincerity, unselfishness, warmth and loyalty to Mommie taught me about what is really important in life. She constantly showed that loving others with true commitment is the best gift you can give another—whether a family member or a friend. Certainly, CC has an excuse to complain or be angry at the world for a childhood totally different from the other children's in her third-grade class. I have never heard her complain about her bald head, swollen face and body (as a result of the steroids), or low energy level, which keeps her from playing outside. CC continues to live her life the way she chooses, and that includes giving of herself to make the world a better place for others, especially Mommie.

CC reminds me to not take those people I love for granted and to look beyond the superficiality that is often found in day-to-day living. I am reminded to be more thankful for what I have today and to not dwell on what is behind me or what lies ahead. CC, just like many other cancer patients, is a true example that we aren't always dealt the perfect hand, so we have to make the best of what we have today.

Anne C. Washburn

Manuel Garcia

Manuel Garcia, a proud youthful father
Was known on his block as a hardworking man.
With a wife and a family, a job and a future
He had everything going according to plan.

One day Manuel Garcia, complaining of stomach pains
Went to the clinic to find the cause.
His body was found to have cancerous tissue
Ignoring the order of natural laws.

So Manuel Garcia of Milwaukee County
Checked into the medical complex in town.
Suddenly seeing his 39 years
Like the sand in an hourglass plummeting down.

"What are my choices?" cried Manuel Garcia.
"You've basically two," was the doctor's decree.
"Your cancer untreated will quickly be fatal,
But treatment is painful with no guarantees. . . ."

And so it began, Manuel's personal odyssey—
Long sleepless nights in a chemical daze
With echoes of footsteps down long lonely corridors
Tolling his minutes and hours away.

With the knowledge that something inside was consum-
  ing him
Manuel Garcia was filled with despair.
He'd already lost 40 pounds to the cancer,
And now to the drugs he was losing his hair.

After nine weeks in treatment the doctor came calling,
Said, "Manuel, we've done about all we can do.
Your cancer could go either way at this juncture;
It's out of our hands and it's now up to you."

He looked in the mirror, a sad frightened stranger
So pale, so wrinkled, so lonely, so scared.
Diseased, isolated, and feeling unlovable—
One-hundred-twenty-six pounds and no hair.

He dreamed of his Carmen at 60 without him,
His four little children not having their Dad,
Of Thursday night card games at Julio's,
And everything else he'd not done that he wished that
  he had.

Awakened from sleep on the day of his discharge
By shuffling feet going all around his bed,
Manuel opened his eyes and thought he was still
  dreaming—
His wife, and four friends with no hair on their heads.

He blinked and he looked again, not quite believing
The four shiny heads all lined up side by side.
And still to that point not a word had been spoken,
But soon they were laughing so hard that they cried.

And the hospital hallways were ringing with voices.
"Patron, we did this for you," said his friends.
And they wheeled him out to the car they had borrowed
"Amigo, estamos contigo, ves . . ."

So Manuel Garcia returned to his neighborhood
Dropped off in front of his two-bedroom flat.
And the block seemed unusually deserted for Sunday;
He drew a deep breath and adjusted his hat.

But before he could enter the front door flew open.
Manuel was surrounded with faces he knew—
Fifty-odd loved ones and friends of the family
With clean-shaven heads and the words "We love you!"

And so Manuel Garcia, a person with cancer,
A father, a husband, a neighbor, a friend,
With a lump in his throat said, "I'm not one for speeches,
But here I have something that needs to be said.

"I felt so alone with my baldness and cancer.
Now you stand beside me, thank Heaven above.
For giving me strength that I need may God Bless you,
And long may we live with the meaning of love.

"For giving me strength that I need may God Bless you,
And long may we live with the meaning of love."

David Roth

Hairs

Everybody in our family has different hair. My papa's hair is short. He doesn't have much, but it suits him. And me, my hair is long and straight. Not a curl if I try. Just straight down past my shoulders. Jeff's hair is great. It is thick and soft. It has body and can be shaped. Very different from my dad's hair now, but it was once the same.

But my mother's hair, my mother's, well it's not really hair. She has cancer so she lost it all. It's growing back, though, and so soft. Like fur. Fuzzy. Soft to touch and soft to the face when she's holding you and you feel safe, it is the warm smell of a baby, it is the smell of comfort when you cuddle up next to her, and she tickles your back letting you know she loves you. All your worries and troubles disappear when she holds you. When I rub her head it is like rubbing a magic lamp. I wish for her to be happy and healthy, and for all her beautiful hair to come back to protect and keep her head warm the way she protects and keeps me warm. That's Mama's hair, like a baby. Soft and warm like her heart.

Jaime Rosenthal

Dear Mommy

Dear mommy;
I love you I wush you could stay with
me but you have to get better
it was good that you came down
and saw all you freinds I will be
still calling you every night before
I go to bed. you are the best mother
any kid can have and I love you.
sooooo much Miss. Grant say's hi too
and so does Miss. Zagger and
Mr. Halleday every body says Hi. you
will get drugs and you will get better
soon and come home to us and
all your freinds.

Your pal
Alexi

Saint Christopher's Protection

Dear Jacqueline:

When you read this letter, it will be Father's Day. I want to tell you a wonderful story about your dad. He is a pretty private person and I'm afraid he might never tell you himself. It is a story that you should know—and perhaps one day pass on to your children.

Your father and I had been friends for years. On a hot August day in 1992 in Boise, Idaho, I met him for lunch. You see, I had cancer and was leaving to begin the long process of a bone marrow transplant at Stanford University Hospital. I was optimistic, but bone marrow transplants are dangerous procedures. It was possible that I would never see your father again and I wanted to tell him good-bye. I was only 39 when I was diagnosed with non-Hodgkin's lymphoma, an unusual cancer for someone so young. Worse yet, the only course of treatment at the time of the original diagnosis was chemotherapy for the rest of my life, which at best would have been only 10 years longer.

The doctors at Stanford determined that I had potential

as a bone marrow transplant candidate. It was a possible cure, but my cancer didn't fit the standard treatment regimen. After hours of uncomfortable tests, difficult discussions and refusal of coverage by my insurance company, I was still determined that I would have that transplant! With my whole heart and soul I tried to convince the Stanford doctors that I could be an exceptional patient. They finally agreed, but they had to write a new protocol, just for me. Yes, I was going to have a bone marrow transplant!

Your dad was pretty shocked to see me when I showed up for our lunch. A brunette with naturally curly hair, I showed up that day with a blond page-boy. It was a wig to cover up the hair I had lost after seven months of chemotherapy. Instead of trying to find a wig that matched my natural hair, I had the page-boy style that I had always wanted in high school. Facing cancer taught me to take risks and try new things. I had learned that life is short and that I should follow my dreams. "Later" might be too late.

Over our meal, the two of us laughed about stories from the past and talked about my terrifying present and unknown future. As you can imagine, it was saying good-bye that I dreaded. As we stood on the sidewalk in front of my car, your dad reached into his pocket and handed me an envelope. Immediately, the words "Saint Christopher medal" flashed into my mind, and I don't know why because neither he nor I am Catholic. He said, "This is for you, but don't open it until you are on the airplane bound for California." He kissed me on the cheek and was gone.

Two days later, shortly after take-off, I opened that envelope. It was, indeed, a Saint Christopher medal—a very special one. On one side of the silver pendant was the U.S. Army's emblem and on the other, Saint Christopher. Your father's enclosed note to me read:

Dear Cindy,

Although I am not famous for my willingness to open up and express my feelings, I want you to know that you are a very special friend. My mom gave me this Saint Christopher medal when I went to Vietnam. She assured me it would keep me safe, and it did. Someday I would like to pass it on to my daughter, Jacqueline, but right now it has a more important use. Please take it and I give you assurance: it will keep you safe. Believe that everything you are going through will be worth it for the long term.

All the best,
Jim

I cried. I was afraid, very afraid, as your dad must also have been when he went off to war, but now I knew I had another reason to believe I would survive. I wore the Saint Christopher medal from that moment on.

My transplant was exceptionally difficult. I suffered severe side effects. The radiation I endured was said to be the equivalent of having been a mile from a nuclear explosion; a dangerous fungus lingered on my lungs. High-dose chemotherapy caused second-degree burns on my hands and feet. My body was so affected that you would never have recognized me: I looked like a monster.

Early signs of transplant success were shattered the day after I left the hospital. My transplant had failed. The combined reasons for the transplant's failure put me in a unique category—what happened to me happens to only 1 percent of transplant patients. There were no options but a stem-cell rescue, an uncertain procedure that might re-infuse my own cancer cells. I faced death square in the face in the weeks I waited for the second transplant to engraft. I was in the hospital for 54 days. I had left Boise on August

14, 1992, and returned home three months later, on December 5. In February, a blood clot, a residual from transplant, passed through my heart but did not harm me. I had experienced miracles. I was lucky to be alive.

As I write this letter, nearly four years have gone by and I am still cancer-free. Your father was right: Saint Christopher protected me.

I remember now that your father had seen a lot of action as a platoon leader and first lieutenant in the infantry. Although he never considered himself a hero, he distinguished himself by earning a bronze star for valor and a purple heart—he was wounded in action on the day two of his good friends died.

Your father wore his medal with faith, Jacqueline—and so did I. When it becomes yours one day, I hope you and your children will remember its history and the stories of courage and friendship that it has to tell.

All my love,
Cindy

Cynthia Bonney Mannering

Our Hero Brian

What is it like for an 18-year-old high school senior to find out that he has two inoperable pineal brain tumors? *Am I going to die? Why me? Why now?* These were just some of the questions that ran through our son Brian's mind.

For two months we didn't know what was happening to our son—he lost weight, wasn't eating and was not himself. He withered away right before our eyes from 140 pounds to 120 pounds in a month, for no apparent reason.

After complaining of double vision, an MRI of the brain was taken and the tumors discovered. We were all shocked, but it answered our question as to why he had the anorectic symptoms.

After the initial shock, Brian had a few days of ups and downs accepting and understanding what really happened as well as the treatment that lay ahead.

Radiation treatments began right after Christmas and with a positive attitude, he surprised us all and sailed through them. Despite being a little tired, he continued going to school every day. His classmates and teachers were amazed.

After the treatments ended he started practicing with

the varsity basketball team. He was able to play a few minutes in a few games just before the season ended, and they were momentous occasions. Just seeing him on the court brought tears and cheers from everyone in the stands who knew what he had been through. Thanks to a very understanding coach (whose wife had breast cancer), he was able to stay on the team throughout the season. At the end-of-season banquet, he was presented the Coaches Award because of the inspiration he showed his teammates, whether at practice or supporting them at their games. Though times were tough, he never gave up. He gave 110 percent of his time and energy.

Then chemotherapy started for five consecutive days, then on days nine and 16 again, for four months. Hair loss, fatigue, poor appetite and constipation were some of the "minor" complications he suffered. These he took in stride and tried to work around them.

During this time an older family friend was diagnosed with lung cancer. Because of Brian's great outlook he was able to talk to our friend, sharing encouragement through rough times.

He attended school for three out of four weeks a month during this time. Amazingly, he kept up with his studies with the help of understanding teachers, friends and the school psychologist. Though he missed some important senior events because of chemotherapy, he graduated with his class with distinguished honors! He was surprised when he was selected the Most Inspirational Male Athlete of the year.

Summer vacation was a welcomed change for Brian as well as the whole family. It was a time for kicking back, having fun and feeling good. We spent a month in Hawaii relaxing and visiting friends and relatives. Now Brian is looking forward to a fresh start this fall at UCLA!

Our family has been through a lot together, but Brian

showed us that with perseverance, no matter how devastating the situation is, it can be conquered. His positive attitude and constant smile, day after day despite enduring painful, frightening situations, made us all very proud of him. I know he has grown a lot through this experience and is ready to face the world.

Brian, we wish you happiness and success in everything you do. Remember: Mom, Dad and sister Amy will always be here for you. We love you!

Norma Yamamoto

Happy Anniversary

Seven days without laughter make one weak.

Joel Goodman

My father-in-law, who was suffering from brain cancer, came home from a hospital stay. It was his and my mother-in-law's anniversary, so I suggested that they invite a few friends over for dinner.

Jimmy managed to get out of bed to join us. The strain of feeding himself and the presence of guests were obviously tiring him. Knowing that he could not hear very well, my mother-in-law passed a note to me to give to him. I read it and laughed hysterically. She remembered what she wrote and laughed, too.

The note said, "Happy Anniversary, dear. Do you want to go to bed?"

Jimmy read his wife's note, looked across the table, and with a twinkle in his eye and a smile on his face said, "I would love to, dear, but we have company."

Allen Klein
from The Healing Power of Humor

Love and Support

On October 1, 1994, I met the man who became the most important person in my life. On Thursday, October 20, 1994, I was diagnosed with non-Hodgkin's lymphoma.

Terry, my husband, and I met through the personal ads of our local paper. We talked for a week prior to meeting. We could not immediately meet because I was feeling so ill. So on Saturday, October 1, we met at a nearby park and hiked while talking for hours. We were instant friends. Throughout the next couple of weeks, I saw an ear, nose and throat specialist for what doctors thought was a sinus infection. On Thursday, October 13, I was referred to a cancer specialist, who immediately checked me into a hospital. I was terrified; I was only 30, had only been teaching first grade for three years, and had never been married. I felt as though this could not possibly be happening to me. I was too young and always healthy. I called my new friend and in tears told him that I would be in the hospital for a couple of days. I begged Terry to consider keeping our friendship, but I would have understood if he simply stopped calling. Terry said he would be at the hospital that evening; I had my doubts. True to his word, Terry came to the hospital at 7:00 P.M., with a stuffed koala bear in hand. Terry came to the hospital every night that week. On Thursday, October 20, I received my diagnosis and was told I could not return to school for four months. That evening I asked my new friend whatever would I do for four months and he responded. "Plan a wedding?" Thus began the most terrifying, painful and exciting period of my life.

Throughout the chemotherapy, which left me nauseous and weak, Terry sat with me, discussing the wedding plans and helping me to focus on the happy and hopefully cancer-free future.

On January 21, 1995, Terry and I were married. Three days later, I went into the hospital for high-dose chemotherapy and a bone marrow transplant.

For three weeks (10 days of which I was in an isolation room), Terry came to the hospital and slept over when he could. When the pain and depression got the best of me, I concentrated on my new husband and all of the different things we would do together. I planned a family dinner for a month after release from the hospital and I thought about the menu and how my relatives would be around me and I would feel surrounded by their support and love.

Each day throughout my hospital stay, my mother sat with me. She asked the doctors questions I was too drugged or too sick to ask for myself. Mom talked when I felt up to it and cross-stitched when I was sleeping. For a large portion of each day, either my mother or my husband sat with me and helped me through the toughest times.

I have now been in remission for six months. I credit my recovery to a wonderful man who saw beyond those ugly cancer cells and to a family whose love and support kept me going on even the most tenuous days.

Christine M. Creley

Love Cures People

We began by imagining that we are giving to them; we end by realizing that they have enriched us.

Pope John Paul II

In August 1992, a beautiful baby girl was born to a very special couple. For the first six months of Paige's life, she cried with colic. Her parents lovingly called her their "baby from hell."

She was a beautiful child, with big brown eyes, and you couldn't help but fall in love with her. On her first birthday, Paige climbed up on my lap and my heart was hers forever.

In March 1995, I received a frantic phone call from Paige's mom, telling me that Paige was diagnosed with cancer and that they were on their way to Children's Hospital in Los Angeles.

As the days went by, the news grew more and more grim. I called everyone I knew and asked them to start a prayer chain.

Paige battled that monster first with chemotherapy,

then radiation, and finally a bone marrow transplant that took place in early October 1995.

Through it all, this amazing three-year-old remained cheerful and gentle as ever. She won the hearts of doctors and nurses alike. Paige's mom never left her side and believed that if she just loved Paige enough, Paige would be okay.

October 31, 1995, Halloween, our Paige came home for good. We had the miracle for which we all prayed. The doctors were amazed at her quick response to her treatments, but her positive attitude amazed them even more.

They weren't alone in this amazement. I had been collecting surprises for Paige over the months she was hospitalized, waiting for the day I could watch her open the bag full of gifts.

As she opened the magical bag of surprises, Paige discovered that several of the toys were ones she already had. I suggested to her mom that she could take them back and exchange them for something she didn't have. I heard Paige's soft little voice ask her mom if they could put these toys in the Christmas bin in front of one of the local stores so that other children could enjoy them. The pride on her mom's face said it all.

At that moment, I realized the power that love has. Love cures people, both the giver and the receiver.

Janine Crawford

Out in the Open

I had two brain operations before I came to a meeting at The Wellness Community* on the topic of "The Family and Cancer." There were about 25 other cancer patients and their families. I was 29, and my mother, father and sister came with me. We all lived together. During that meeting, I started talking about the second operation and how terribly frightened I was that the cancer would reappear, and I started to cry. I hadn't talked about my fear with my family because I didn't want them to be frightened, too. When my mother saw my tears, she took me in her arms as she did when I was a very little girl, and we sat there crying together. My father and sister moved closer and we all held hands. They told me later they didn't want to intrude. My mother, still holding me tight, said she had always known about my fear because the entire family was worried about the same thing, but that they didn't want me to worry about them. So now it was out in the open. We loved each other and we were all too frightened to talk to each other and now we could talk about anything.

Michelle

---

* You can contact The Wellness Community by writing 2716 Ocean Park Blvd., Suite 1040, Santa Monica, CA 90405, or calling (310) 314-2555. Also, we recommend you read *The Wellness Community: Guide to Fighting for Recovery from Cancer* by Harold H. Banjamin, Ph.D. New York: G.P. Putnam's Sons, 1995.

"You Are Going to Need a Surgeon"

"You are going to need a surgeon."

With those words, I began a four-year roller coaster ride, both plunging into fear and soaring with hope. The diagnosis was colon cancer; the statistics, 55 percent death rate. But at least I finally knew why I was so tired that even lifting a jigsaw puzzle piece took more energy than I could muster.

Yet one of the hardest tasks in winning my battle came right at the beginning. Somewhat in shock, I left my diagnostician, met with the surgeon he recommended, agreed to enter the hospital in four days, and went home. That was the easy part. The difficult part was finding a way to tell my family . . . and, especially, to tell my husband, Norm, who was 3,000 miles away on a three-month contract. Even as a child, I had always been the healthy one in the family. Besides that, it was two weeks before Christmas. How, then, to tell them that not only was I not well (a quaint euphemism), but that there was a very strong possibility I could die?

I never did find the words. Instead, my later-to-be-psychologist daughter, Nicole, finally commented that I looked odd; then, remembering I had been to the doctor, guessed that he gave me bad news. She also took on the job I was totally incapable of, that of telling her father.

Norm is one of those type-A-in-super-bold people. By the time I entered the hospital four days later, he had wound up his contract, packed for his move back home, arranged for my mother to come, discovered three alternate treatments and had people in two churches praying for my recovery . . . not bad for one weekend's work.

In the meantime, my almost-grown kids, Noral, Kal and Nicole, put on brave faces and exuded extra energy attempting to pretend that we were decorating our two-story Christmas tree (an engineering feat in its own right), just like we did every year. None of us knew quite what to expect or what to do about it.

But after my surgery, my children, along with their father, our Jaycee Senator friends and about 500 members of our professional association, the National Speakers Association (NSA), soon figured it out . . . I was a little slower.

My family first descended on the hospital with most of the Christmas decorations from our oversized home. These soon festooned every available wall, every bed rail and even my catheter hose. I had chosen to go into a public ward in order to have company. I had company. Every nurse, doctor, candy striper and housekeeper, along with a string of patients, came by to see this splash of color and frivolity in the serious atmosphere of the surgery wing.

Christmas morning, the traffic to my window was constant, when sons Kal, my early-bird designer, and Noral, always calm in a crisis, braved the pre-dawn cold of an Ottawa December to erect in the snow of the hospital yard a 12-foot sign, on which the family had painted "Merry Christmas, Mom."

My operation had been a few days before, on December 21, and the news was mixed: the tumor was out, but it had been large. While I was, thankfully, not given chemotherapy or radiation, my surgeon, Dr. Doubek, promised me no more than two years to live.

The news moved quickly. The amount and the depth of just sheer caring that poured from across the continent was a wonderful shock. You see, one of the horrible things about cancer is the enormous loss of your self-worth. I truly believe that unless a person who has the disease regains the feeling that he or she really matters, the person will die.

When all the cards and calls arrived, along with messages that people were having their church congregations pray for me, I reached a stage where I would honestly have felt I was letting people down if I died . . . especially Big E. Larry Moles from Lima, Ohio, who took two trips to the border to get a teddy bear as large as himself (now known as Larr Bear) through Canadian customs. We later decided customs people figured he was using the bear as a camouflage for drugs or other contraband. Officials seem suspicious of just plain friendship.

"Friendship" is one item I place on my "must have" list as part of my own growth out of cancer. My first step was to simplify my life by determining what was truly important to me . . . and shedding what was not. It is amazing how short one's "must have" list really is! Try your own list one day when you are feeling overwhelmed—it may change your future.

There is a lot of discussion about the role of positive thinking in curing disease. For me, there is no question. It works.

It works, that is, if you work at it. Positive thinking to cure yourself of physical illness, or of life's negative strokes, goes well beyond thinking positive thoughts. My struggle with cancer took four years and several operations . . . but I am now, 10 years later, officially a cancer survivor. Now, each time I hit a bad patch, I tap into the same two elements that pulled me up during the crisis: love from family and friends, and a consistent use of my mind to heal my body—cell by cell, through concentration and visualization.

I continue to stretch my mind for health and to "keep on track" with my life. Each of us can do this for ourselves. Yet, as my husband often quotes, "No man (person, in today's vernacular) is an island." Equally significant to our health and well-being are the Pat Balls of the world who wrote to me that she was concerned about intruding, but just felt she had to let me know she cared. Caring we cannot do just for ourselves, it grows when it's shared with others . . . and it can save lives.

Delva Seavy-Rebin

I Believe in Miracles

In order to be a realist you must believe in miracles.

David Ben-Gurion

"Chris is dying. I'm going to sell his car." Easter, 1989. My ex-husband was on the phone talking about our 25-year-old son. I was more than stunned, but also very angry!

I knew that Chris hadn't been feeling well—"a stomach virus" is the way he described it. But since it kept getting worse, he went to the hospital, where the prognosis was far from positive. In the doctor's words, "The bad news is that your son has lymphoma—the fastest growing cancer. The good news is that it is a cancer that responds well to chemotherapy—once we stabilize his condition, that is."

For six weeks, that is exactly what the Cleveland Clinic attempted to do, as Chris remained in the intensive care unit on a respirator. His condition deteriorated to the point that the first day I visited him, I walked right past his bed. I didn't even recognize my own son!

It wasn't time for him to die. He had too much living still to do. I decided to put to work all of the visualization techniques I had learned, to call up my power of positive thinking and to maintain my natural optimism. I told my ex-husband—who was already receiving sympathy cards from his group of negative friends—that I believe in miracles. Chris would pull through. He mustn't sell Chris' car.

I don't know if you've ever experienced the intensive care unit in a hospital. It isn't a pleasant place to visit. There are all sorts of bells and whistles. Nurses and doctors are rushing to answer alarms. The patients are swollen and possess a deathly pallor. Negativity is in the air. I even had a doctor say to me, "Don't you realize how sick your son is? How can you be so positive?" I had him taken off the case.

We were only allowed 15 minutes twice a day. I went every morning. And every morning I took Chris' hand and told him to visualize summer, with the warm weather, the sun and the flowers (all of which he loved). I noticed that every time I visited, a certain light came on and a beep sounded. The nurses told me that it indicated that while I was there, Chris breathed on his own so the respirator reacted. I knew we were making progress.

Chris recovered enough to come home for the summer, still on chemotherapy, with short stays back at the clinic. Together, we listened to tapes, we talked about the future, we concentrated on the beauty of every moment. By December, he was in total remission. They called it a miracle.

In April of 1990, he elected to undergo a bone marrow transplant as a preventive measure. This spring, we celebrated his fifth anniversary of remission. Yes, I do believe in miracles!

Chris King

6

ON SUPPORT

The most important medicine is tender love and care.

Mother Teresa

"Pete, You Have Cancer!"

In the fall of 1992, I was driving back to my office from an important lunch in downtown Vancouver when the phone rang in the car. I've had a phone in the car for quite a while, but it still amazes me that you can actually be called and make calls from a car!

It was my doctor.

"Pete," he said. "I don't know what you're doing right now, but you need to come to my office immediately."

"What's the matter?"

On a car phone!

I pulled off to the side of the road and cried. Rolling tears. And between the tears, my life, every important moment I had ever lived, rolled too, like a great screen before me. Cancer! The terrifying words I just heard triggered all kinds of levers and emotions that most of the time were inactively just there. Now, like circuit breakers snapping into life at a hydro substation, they were part of terrifying real time.

Without a doubt, I was going to die. Done. Finished. And with approaching death, my value system, my roots, my life's foundations were about to be tested as never before. My proclaimed faith was on the line.

But we humans come around. The survival instinct cuts in. Severely beaten, but already feeling hints of reserve strength, I immediately wondered if I could perhaps overcome whatever it was I now had. Could I be as positive as I tell people in speeches and seminars around the world that I am? Could I impact my own life as I've been told I impact the lives of others?

When I called my doctor back, he told me to pick up my wife and come to his office. Kay was home from her studies and the two of us went hand in hand to see my doctor.

"A simple operation," he said in his best airline pilot voice. "Six to eight stitches and about 20 minutes. We're going to take a piece from your butt and use it to patch your face." Interesting. My backside suddenly felt exposed!

They took me into the hospital, laid me down and covered my face. It wasn't that simple. It took them 18 needles just to freeze the area of my face where the restoration was to happen. I had no idea what was going on except that so far nothing was happening to my rear end. There had obviously been a change in plan. The cancer would be removed in some other way.

An hour-and-a-half and 125 stitches later—with a huge, heart-shaped, puffy, still-bleeding scar on my face—I said to Eric, the plastic surgeon who performed this neat piece of work: "So what have you done?"

"It's a new procedure that I learned a couple of weeks ago in Paris," he said. "I thought I'd try it out on you."

"Thanks heaps," I said.

Eric told me that despite the initial blood and gore, the scar would heal. In a few months I would be very happy, and in a year or so, the scar would be all but invisible. The V-flap operation, he said, would be much better in the long run than affixing the skin from my rear, which because of its unique pigmentation would remain forever "butt white."

Round One appeared to be a success, but a bigger test was yet to come. The medical team was not 100 percent sure that they had removed all of the cancer. I had to go to the Vancouver Cancer Clinic for further examination by a 10-doctor team, a conference to determine whether or not a second operation was required. The thought of it was terrifying.

I should tell you right now that despite a constant, not-too-enthusiastic fight against flab, I have really enjoyed a healthy life. No hospitals, except to visit others; no operations, no anesthetics. Another operation, I quickly concluded, would introduce me to everything all at once. I might never be the same again. Worse than that, I would probably die. Again, my mind skidded me straight to the morgue!

Whoa there, Pete! How about the skills of the doctors? The technology? We all have special talents, don't we? Could it be that whatever they have in store for you has been done quite successfully hundreds of times to others? The surgical fight against cancers of all kinds has seen many incredible victories. Where's your faith and positive attitude? How about the love that's pouring out for you from your family and friends?

The doctors decided that the second operation was indeed required, and they set the date for seven-and-a-half hours of surgery at Vancouver General Hospital.

Charlie Trimbell, who is president of Oppenheimer Bros.—one of Western Canada's leading food brokers—and is a good friend, told me, "Pete, you have pretty good people skills. When you get into the hospital, put them into overdrive. Use your skills to get on the good side of everyone who comes into your room. Regardless of what they do, learn their names and try to find out what they do. It will be the beginning of greater understanding at an incredibly important time. The care you receive from doctors, nurses and orderlies will be gentler because you will give each of them something of yourself." I told him I would do my best.

I took in two boxes of my first book, *How to Soar with the Eagles,* and gave them away at every opportunity. No matter who came into my room, they got a signed copy of my book. Was I covering my aforementioned backside? You never know, do you?

As well as making all these literary presentations, I talked at length to all of the people involved in my immediate hospital world, and to all those who would play a role in my surgery the following day.

I paid special attention to the anesthetist. Len was a warm, friendly, efficient and sensitive man from England. When he came to see me on the eve of my operation, I spent more time questioning him than all of the doctors and nurses together. I told Len that in the morning, just before he put me under, I wanted to gather all of the nurses and doctors around my bed and offer them a five-minute Legge motivational speech. Some last-minute insurance.

"Really?" said Len. "And what are you going to say?"

"What will I say? I will say: You doctors and nurses do this operation almost every day of every week. You are considered the best in Western Canada. You probably view this as just another neck dissection on just another body, but I'd like to tell you that for me, this is the first and only time I'm going to have this operation. Today, you will be better in all of your functions than you have ever been before. Your skills will be superb. No side effects whatsoever. No mistakes. Just a smooth, well-performed, 100 percent successful operation, the best you can possibly perform." I used every adjectival rouser in the book, my own and everyone else's!

"Great," said Len. "I'm looking forward to it."

The next morning at five, my nurse awakened me, and, not surprisingly, gave me pills to make me sleep. Then it was onto the trolley and off to the O.R. In there, all kinds of people scurried around, checking equipment, doing whatever it is that these green-gowned creatures do. Sharpening knives? Recovering from the night before?

I looked at the clock. It was 8:10 A.M. Time for the motivational. "Okay," said Len. "Just one minor adjustment before you begin . . . " and as he spoke, a world of nothingness closed around me.

I looked at the clock again. It was 8:15. Five minutes later. Nope. It was twelve hours and five minutes later. I was no longer surrounded by the twilight of morning. There was pain, and a great city hospital went about its business in the darkness of a winter evening. The deed had been done. Things would be different, but I was very much alive.

Alive, but not necessarily the happiest of campers. Christmas was coming, and I knew that in this season of traditional celebration, when families invariably came closer together, I would stand out as a substantially scarred face in the family crowd. My cheek was swathed in dressings, but I knew that beneath it all was a different-looking husband, a different-looking dad, a different-looking guy who would appear at future bookings on the podiums of the world. Different looking and substantially broken inside.

Would there even be future bookings? I asked myself. *Maybe I'd lost it.* I tested my voice and it was little more than a croak. I moved in the darkness and several I.V.'s followed me around, tugging painfully at my flesh. *Could I ever swing a golf club again?* I doubted it.

A lot of people have trouble visiting the sick in hospitals, especially those who come out looking different than when they went in. Visitors have to steel themselves for these visits: attempt to disregard the smells, the foreign images. They have to say to themselves: "I'm going in here to make this person feel better, and no matter what I'm about to see in that bed, I won't flinch."

My family came early to see me, and Kay and my three daughters all flinched. They caught themselves quickly, but they flinched. I'd never hold that against them. It's just one of those things that happens when you're shocked by an image you weren't expecting. I suspect that I looked pretty awful.

My eldest daughter, Samantha, dived in for the kill—and I'll always be grateful that she did. I can't remember her exact words, but whatever they were, she got them right.

"For years, Dad, you've talked about people who end up in situations like this, people who have been bruised and beaten, who, for whatever reason, are hurt physically or mentally in life. And what you have said to them is that they must live for today and have hope for tomorrow. . . . "

Both of us had tears in our eyes.

"Yes," I said.

"Now it's your turn to be the model. Now it's your turn to dig deep and draw on all of those things that you've said are important in life—courage, hope, love, the strength of the family. We'll be with you. No matter what."

Pete Legge

Teens Launch Campaign to Save Dying Baby's Life

As he left home for his teaching job at Kamiakin Junior High, near Seattle, Washington, on February 26, 1992, Jeff Leeland prayed for his son, Michael. The six-month-old boy had undergone hospital tests, and results were due that day.

In January, Michael had developed pneumonia; tests revealed that the clotting cells in his blood were at a surprisingly low level. He was referred to Children's Hospital and Medical Center.

At 10 o'clock, Jeff called home. "Hello, sweetheart . . . what's wrong? Michael has what?" Through tears, Jeff's wife, Kristi, repeated the diagnosis: "Michael has myelodysplasia syndrome. It's a pre-leukemia disease." Kristi's voice broke. "He needs a bone marrow transplant."

Jeff felt as though a sledgehammer had slammed into his gut.

Later, Kristi and Jeff shared the news with their other children: Jaclyn, nine, Amy, six, and Kevin, three. The family members were to have their blood tested in the hope that one of them would be an eligible bone marrow donor.

On March 20, Kristi called Jeff at work. Her elated voice cried out, "Amy's a perfect match!" It was the couple's first taste of tangible hope.

Unexpectedly, however, a dark cloud cast its shadow over this hope. The Leelands' insurance policy had a 12-month waiting period on benefits relating to organ transplants. Jeff had signed up for the coverage the previous October.

A bone marrow transplant costs $200,000, money the family didn't have. On top of this, the transplant needed to be done soon.

In solitude, one May morning, Jeff lay bare his wounded soul. Writing in his journal, his words formed a prayer to God, his only hope. His little boy was dying. In the stillness, a deep calming came in a whisper to his soul. God has everything in control.

Several days later, Dameon Sharkey, one of Jeff's students, walked in. At 13, with learning difficulties and few friends, Dameon faced his own mountains of adversity. The teen approached Jeff and gave him his life savings— twelve $5 bills. After hugging and thanking Dameon, Jeff went to the principal's office. They agreed to use Dameon's gift to establish "The Michael Leeland Fund."

From then on, the Leelands witnessed the incredible difference kids can make. In the coming weeks, the high-spirited junior high kids staged a walkathon, held a raffle and pursued media contacts. The ninth-grade class donated the proceeds from its dance to Michael. Mary, an eighth-grade student, cashed in $300 in savings bonds. Jon, a ninth-grader, knocked on doors in his neighborhood. The Leelands were awestruck by this outpouring of love.

As a result of the students' appeal, reports appeared in the local media. After reading about Michael, a man walked into the bank with a check for $10,000, and a second-grade girl donated the contents of her piggy bank.

Just one week after Dameon's gift, Michael's account grew to $16,000.

One woman set up phone chains for prayer and support all over the state. One man, though jobless and $35,000 in debt, sent $10 because "I have my health."

Four weeks after Dameon's gift opened the floodgates, the fund totaled over $220,000. Michael would get a second chance.

In July, the boy endured 12 days of chemotherapy and radiation to destroy his diseased marrow before doctors transfused his sister's healthy cells into him. On Michael's first birthday, his family received great news: Michael's white cell count had finally exceeded the minimum acceptable level! A week later, Michael was able to go home.

Today, three years later, the disease is in remission. Doctors say Michael has a 95 percent probability of a lifetime cure.

The Leelands pray that the compassion their community demonstrated will not die out, and that Michael will one day be as selfless as Dameon Sharkey, the boy whose gift started Michael's life-saving fund, and who became a vital link in a chain of love.*

Jeff Leeland

---

* The Leeland family has now established The Sparrow Foundation, a nonprofit organization that provides seed money to youth groups involved in fund-raising efforts. For more information, write to: The Sparrow Foundation, 1155 N. 130th, Suite 310, Seattle, WA 98133.

Judy

Judy started chemotherapy just prior to attending one of my workshops for the first time. Although it was necessary for friends to drive her to and from her treatments and stay with her afterward, she felt that she was imposing on them. Because of these feelings, as well as the rigors of the chemotherapy, she desperately needed love and support. Many workshop participants felt rejected while growing up and were eager to shower love on a recipient they knew wouldn't refuse it. It was a powerful healing process. The group bonded quickly, and I decided to keep the group dynamic going by meeting monthly.

At the next workshop, Judy lightheartedly shared her experiences about losing her hair, which she said was now falling out by the handful. "Maybe I should get a Mohawk hairdo and dye it purple. I might as well have fun with this," she said. Her courageous attitude was an inspiration to us all. She shrugged this off, saying, "People are resilient in different areas. I just happen to have a lot of resiliency in this area."

She never did get a Mohawk, but she did start wearing caps—some had sequins; a favorite one had a propeller.

One day, she called me just as I was leaving for the December workshop. "I had chemo yesterday, and I'm just too nauseous to make it," she said. At the workshop, we made a special tape for her with messages from group members. When I told her about it, she cried.

After three months of being unable to attend the group workshop, Judy let us know that she would once again grace us with her presence. When she walked in the room, we engulfed her with our hugs. Left unspoken was our concern for her emotional state; it's one thing to joke about your hair falling out, and another to actually experience it. We wondered how she had stood up under the strain.

Judy answered our question when she sat down and removed her scarf. I choked back my tears and then burst into laughter as I read the words on her bald head: "And you think *you're* having a bad hair day!"

Nancy Richard-Guilford

Mrs. G in 3B

The notice was posted next to the tenants' mailboxes in the apartment building I'd just moved into in Brooklyn, New York. "A Mitzvah for Mrs. Green," it read. "Sign up to drive Mrs. G in #3B home from her chemotherapy treatments twice a month."

Since I wasn't a driver, I couldn't add my name, but the word mitzvah lingered in my thoughts after I went upstairs. It's a Hebrew word that means "to do a good deed," or "an act that expresses God's will." It is more than that, really, more like a commandment to do things for others.

And according to my grandmother, it also had another meaning. This was the one she was always pointing out to me because she'd notice how shy I was about letting people do things for me. "Linda, it's a blessing to do a mitzvah for someone else, but sometimes it's a blessing to let another person do something for you."

Grandma would be shaking her head at me right now. Several of my friends at the graduate school I attended nights had offered to help me settle in after the moving men left, but I'd said I could manage. Letting them help would have interfered with my image of myself as a capable and independent woman of 21.

Snowflakes had been tumbling past my window for several hours when it came time to leave for class. I pulled on two sweaters, a coat, a wool hat and boots, bundling up for the trek to the bus stop that the real estate agent had dismissed as a short stroll. Maybe in May it was a stroll, but in this December storm it was a hike. As I topped off my outfit with a blue scarf that Grandma had crocheted for me, I could almost hear her voice: "Why don't you see if you can find a lift?"

A thousand reasons why popped into my head: I don't know my neighbors; I don't like to impose; I feel funny asking for favors. Pride would not let me knock on a door and say, "It's a 10-minute ride by car but a long wait for the bus, and it's a 30-minute bus ride, so could you possibly give me a lift to school?"

I trudged to the bus stop, reaching it just as a bus went by.

Three weeks later, on the night of my final exam, the snow was falling steadily. I slogged through oceans of slush to the bus stop. For an hour, I craned my neck, praying desperately that a bus would come. Then I gave up. The wind at my back pushed me toward home, as I prayed, *Dear God, how can I get to school? What should I do?*

As I pulled Grandma's scarf more tightly around my neck, again I seemed to hear that whisper: *Ask someone for a lift! It could be a mitzvah.*

That idea had never really made sense to me. And even if I wanted to ask someone for a good deed, which I did not, there wasn't a soul on the street.

But as I shoved the door of my apartment building open, I found myself face to face with a woman at the mailbox. She was wearing a brown coat and had a set of keys in her hand. Obviously she had a car, and just as obviously, she was going out. In that split second, desperation overcame pride, and with my breath coming out in white puffs in the freezing hallway, I blurted, "Could you possibly give me a lift?" I hurriedly explained, ending with, "I never ask anybody for a lift, but . . ."

An odd look crossed the woman's face, and I added, "Oh! I live in 4R. I moved in recently."

"I know," she said. "I've seen you through the window." Then, after an almost imperceptible hesitation, "Of course, I'll give you a lift. Let me get my car key."

"Your car key?" I repeated. "Isn't that it in your hand?"

She looked down. "No, no, I was just going to get my mail. I'll be right back." And she disappeared upstairs, ignoring my "Ma'am! Please! I don't mean to put you out!" I was terribly embarrassed. But when she came back, she spoke so warmly as we plodded our way to a garage across the street that I stopped feeling uncomfortable.

"You know the way better than I," she said. "Why don't you drive?"

"I can't," I said.

Now I felt inept again.

She just laughed and patted me on the hand, saying, "It's not so important," and then I laughed, too.

"You remind me of my grandmother," I said.

At that, a slight smile crossed her lips. "Just call me Grandma Alice. My grandchildren do. And you are . . .?" As she maneuvered her car—one of those big cars, like a tank—down the slushy streets, I introduced myself.

When she dropped me off, I thanked her profusely and stood there waving as she drove away. My final exam was a breeze compared with the ordeal I'd gone through to get to it, and asking Grandma Alice for help had loosened me so that after class I was able to ask easily, "Is anyone going my way?" It turned out that while I'd been waiting for a bus every night, three fellow students passed my apartment house. "Why didn't you say something before?" they chorused.

Back home as I walked up the stairs, I passed Grandma Alice leaving her neighbor's apartment. "Good night, Mrs. Green. See you tomorrow," the neighbor was saying.

I nodded to them and was four steps up the staircase before the name registered in my brain. Mrs. Green. The woman with cancer. "Grandma Alice" was Mrs. Green.

I stood on the stairs, my hand covering my mouth, as the . . . grotesqueness was the only word I could think of . . . of what I had done hit me: I had asked a person struggling with cancer to go out in a snowstorm to give me a lift to school. "Oh, Mrs. Green," I stammered, "I didn't realize who you were. Please forgive me."

I forced my legs to move me up the stairs. In my apartment, I stood still, not taking my coat off. How could I have been so insensitive? In a few seconds, someone tapped on my door. Mrs. Green stood there.

"May I tell you something?" she asked. I nodded slowly, motioning her toward a chair, sinking down onto my couch. "I used to be so strong," she said. She was crying, dabbing at her eyes with a white linen handkerchief. "I used to be able to do for other people. Now everybody keeps doing for me, giving me things, cooking my meals and taking me places. It's not that I don't appreciate it because I do. But tonight before I went out to get my mail, I prayed to God to let me feel like part of the human race again. Then you came along . . ."

Linda Neukrug

The Wellness Community

Though my wife, Harriet, is fine today, in 1972 she had both breasts removed to stop the spread of cancer. Harriet's illness showed me how uniquely destructive cancer is psychologically as well as physically. I also discovered that the emotional distress that accompanies cancer can be almost as debilitating as the illness itself. Because of that realization—and while continuing to practice law in Beverly Hills—I began to study the effect that emotions have on the onset and course of the disease. One of the most important facts I learned is: The belief that everyone with cancer dies of that illness is a dreadful myth. The truth is that there are over 8,000,000 people in the United States today to whom cancer is a memory. This information brings joy and hope to the heart of any person who has ever dreaded the onset of cancer.

My study continued until 1982, when—armed with the information I had gleaned over that 10-year period—I conceived of the Patient Active Concept. The power of the Patient Active Concept awed me. I retired from the practice of law to found The Wellness Community* based on

---

* Harold H. Benjamin, Ph.D., is founder and president of The Wellness Community, Santa Monica, California, and is the author of *The Wellness Community Guide to Fighting for Recovery from Cancer.* For more information call 310-314-2555.

it. I based the Wellness Community Patient Active Concept on the premise that cancer patients don't have to be hopeless, helpless and passive in the face of the illness. There are many actions they can take as partners with their physicians that are likely to improve the quality of their lives, and that may increase the possibility of recovery. Isn't that liberating and empowering? The Wellness Community Patient Active Concept sets forth a series of methods cancer patients can use to join their physician in the fight for recovery: using guided imagery, making plans for the future, controlling stress, avoiding pain, and many others that may have a positive effect on the course of the illness.

The purpose of The Wellness Community was and is to help cancer patients learn what they need to know to fight for their recovery as partners with their physicians. The Wellness Center does this without charging the patient in any way—it is free. Since its founding, over 30,000 participants have used The Wellness Community and over 1,000 physicians have referred their patients to us.

I believe the interaction these people have with each other at The Wellness Community also makes them aware of how much control they have over their lives. They become aware that all of life is a series of choices we must make—whether we want to or not—and that control is not a single act but is a culmination of the decisions we make. It starts with decisions such as, "Taking into account my need for the salary and the insurance my job provides, I will decide whether to remain in this job." If someone has cancer, it may be important to exert control with the following types of decisions: "I will choose what arm the injection will be given into"; "I will choose just how much I will participate in my fight for recovery"; and if the illness becomes desperate, "I will choose how that information will affect me and how I will react to that situation." All of this culminates in the ultimate control: "I know that whatever choice I make will be the correct choice for me."

Harold H. Benjamin, Ph.D.

The Corporate Angel Network

Keyboarding for help on the information super-highway took a new turn this year when a cancer patient posted his SOS on a computer bulletin board and tapped into the Corporate Angel Network (CAN)*, the not-for-profit organization that arranges for cancer patients to use empty seats on company aircraft for transportation to treatment centers across the United States.

Jay Weinberg, CAN Vice President, said an anxious cancer patient posted his inquiry on the nationwide Internet computer network about where to get transportation assistance and was referred to CAN by another Internet subscriber.

And with that one simple listing, one more person joined the ranks of CAN's family of 8,000 cancer patients who have hitched rides aboard corporate jets.

Weinberg partnered with friend Pat Blum 14 years ago to create CAN. Both are recovered cancer patients, Blum from breast cancer 25 years ago and Weinberg from melanoma

---

* You can contact The Corporate Angel Network by writing CAN, Inc., Building One, Westchester Airport, White Plains, NY 10604.

20 years ago. Oddly, both lived within 45 miles of Memorial Sloan-Kettering Cancer Center in New York City and neither endured much of a commute from their homes.

But even though they did not have a difficult commute, they empathize today with what they call "the psychological and emotional journey" cancer patients must take on the road to recovery.

Blum hatched the idea that corporate jets might be able to help shuttle cancer patients when she found herself sitting on a plane waiting on the runway at Westchester County Airport in White Plains, New York, for a number of corporate jets to take off. She noticed that many of them had empty seats.

She phoned Weinberg and they toasted their enterprise over a cup of coffee. That was 14 years ago and in that time, the 8,000-plus CAN cancer patients have been shuttled by 550 participating company aircraft.

Of those, 12 corporations have flown more than 100 patients each. This year, AT&T's 100th flight was nine-year-old Alexis Farrell, who needed a ride from her home in Washington, D.C., to New York, where she was being treated for an autoimmune deficiency.

CAN's youngest rider to date was a 15-day-old infant, Faith Miller, whose journey from hometown Pittsburgh to New York City has also been taken by both her sister and brother, who share her genetic problem.

The oldest cancer patient on CAN so far was Emma Hughes, 93. Despite her age, she drives herself from Phoenix to Scottsdale airport, where she catches the corporate flight to her cancer treatment center in Denver.

As much work that goes into seeing that cancer patients are well taken care of in the air is done on the ground. In CAN's offices at the Westchester County Airport, a full-time staff of three employees is assisted by a battalion of 60 volunteers who help 12 at a time during the five-day-a-week, year-long campaigns to ensure cancer patients get to their treatments.

This year, Blum and Weinberg developed a brochure to inform prospective patients about the service.

Once operated on colored index cards filed in a shoe box, CAN's extensive network of cancer patients and participating corporate aviation departments has been computerized with the help of Weinberg's wife, Marian, who recently updated CAN with a new software program. It is designed to keep track of the data and the flights for life that keep the organization perpetually ready.

The Corporate Angel Network

To Climb a Mountain

Perhaps it was angels. Perhaps it was fate. Perhaps it was just a stroke of luck that led little David to the home of Bob and Doris. Determining how it all happened is just not quite as important as why David's life became so entwined with the couple. In the end the three of them, together, scaled a mountain.

But before David ever came along, before the two teachers ever married, before their love made them increasingly strong, Bob was given six months to live.

Six months. That was it. That's all the time doctors believed he had, once they discovered bone cancer was rotting his arm, a tumor the size of a grapefruit cradled in his left shoulder. The avid surfer, however, didn't believe his destiny was tied to such an early death, and neither did his students. Nearly 100 letters from students, teachers and parents poured in each week while Bob was going through radiation, poked at, x-rayed and given gigantic doses of chemotherapy to shrink his nasty tumor. Despite the pain, despite the surgeries, despite living in a body cast that covered half his body, Bob promised his eighth-grade students at the middle school that he would show up for their graduation at the end of the year. He opted for experimental efforts at UCLA. Rather than having his left arm amputated, they cut out the tumor and hooked in a cadaver's bone up through his shoulder to hold it in place.

This wasn't the first time Bob faced death. He faced it twice before. When he was 16, he was in a terrible car accident that tore away one-third of his face. He was in intensive care for two weeks and had 150 stitches to help rebuild his face. Then he served in Vietnam as an officer and was taking his men off for a mission in a tank, when his supervisor waved him back and told him he was needed. The supervisor traded places with Bob. Leaving without him, the tank was later attacked and exploded, killing all the men inside. And now, he was told he had six months. He just wasn't going to let that happen. "I chose only to live," Bob later said. "It's not about putting your life in order for death. It's not just that. It's doing what you would normally do. Today, I'm going to go to the store. Today, I'm going to go to the theater. Today, I am alive."

Once he had the surgery, Doris and several teachers went to see him, wondering if he could move his arm or ever use it again. He immediately showed them all how useful his arm was. He flipped them off!

He went to the beach every day, and walked in his huge body cast. He learned the art of imaging from The Wellness Community and saw himself only as well. He did as he promised and showed up, body cast and all, at his students' graduation. They dedicated the ceremony to him and he knew he was going to make it—he was a survivor.

In 1983, Doris and Bob's friendship blossomed into love. They married, both at the age of 38, and wanted to have children. They took two paths. Doris tried to get pregnant even though they knew she had endometriosis. And Doris knew they were both capable of adoption. For her, blood lines were secondary in the case of motherhood. She had already raised a young girl from Mexico who was abandoned by her mother. The girl's father had showed up in Doris' English-as-a-Second-Language class with his two children, Olga, 10, and Sotero, 13, in tow. Doris learned their mother had tricked the children into going to the United States to see their father and promised they would come home. But they never did. They moved in with their father and about 20 other people in a small apartment.

Doris couldn't stand it. The more she learned about the family, the more she wanted to help. Olga came into the classes every night crying, longing for her mother. She was afraid. She was in a new country. She didn't know the language. Doris took Olga and Sotero to Disneyland and to the movies. They started coming for dinner and overnight. And finally, Doris suggested to the family that they allow one of the children to move in with her.

"The brother said: 'I'm older and Olga needs a mom,'" Doris recalled. Olga moved right in and Sotero visited nearly every day. It was then—after Doris saw Olga marry and eventually land a job as an assistant teacher in her school—that she knew she could love any child, even if it wasn't her own.

So Doris and Bob devoted their time to adoption efforts while trying to have a child. Many friends and colleagues discouraged the couple from going for a United States adoption. The waiting lines were so long, they were told, and parents change their minds. So they pursued their Latino connections. After all, both spoke Spanish fluently and had lived in Spain. Doris had also lived in Mexico and was quite familiar with the culture.

They put aside money. They attended extensive classes on foreign adoption. They made contacts in Argentina, Panama and Colombia. They networked with people across the United States. They were fingerprinted. They were cleared by the FBI. They wrote 15-page biographies about themselves. They supplied 10 reference letters. And Doris said she learned a great philosophy from one group of parents who adopted: "Don't let one single day go by without doing something toward the adoption process. Then you feel empowered."

The couple decided they didn't care what sex the child was, what race it was or even if he or she had a minor disability. They were willing to adopt right up to the age of four or five.

Every night Doris came home and wondered if she had done something toward the adoption that day.

One evening, she realized she had not asked several doctors she'd known for any help. She sat down and wrote a letter asking an ophthalmologist, an internist and a gynecologist if they could help her and Bob find a baby to adopt. Then one evening at a school open house, the father of two children she had in her classes showed up. He was an orthopedic surgeon. The next day Doris went home and sent him the same letter.

Months went by. They hadn't heard anything. But the international adoption was looking promising. A possibility had arisen in Colombia and they would have to move there for two months to get a child.

A few weeks before they had sent in about $4,000 and their final adoption papers, the phone rang. The wife of an obstetrician was calling and said she'd injured her leg. She went to the orthopedic surgeon that Doris had written to and the surgeon handed her a letter, saying: "Can you do anything for these people?"

The woman knew her husband's practice wasn't in the adoption business. They rarely got involved in anything like that. But hadn't this 17-year-old girl come into the office recently, 38 weeks pregnant, a Catholic who didn't believe in abortion, bringing her mother along? The girl said she knew she was too young and not capable of caring for the child. When the obstetrician's wife returned to the office, she showed her husband the letter. The obstetrician was stunned. He had received three other letters from doctors recommending the same couple. They decided to talk to the girl about Bob and Doris and how four different doctors in the community had highly recommended them as adoptive parents. The girl immediately wanted to meet them.

Doris wasn't so sure. She was scared, scared that once the girl realized Bob had cancer, she wouldn't want them to be the baby's parents. Scared that if she met the girl, she would want to get involved in her life. Being a teacher, all Doris could think about was how she wanted to tutor the girl and help her get a good education. Bob and Doris decided to see if the birth mother would go to counseling if they paid for it. The girl agreed, but as a birth mother, she repeated her request to meet them.

Finally, Doris and Bob agreed. They went to meet her at their lawyer's office. Doris will never forget that day. She stared steadily at the door handle of the office and when it finally turned, in burst this tiny, blonde 17-year-old girl, her hair in a ponytail, bubbling with excitement and energy. The girl, the mother, the attorney, Doris and Bob all sat down in a circle at a large oak table.

The girl looked the couple directly in the eye and said: "I know this is difficult for you. But I decided I had to exercise my rights as the birth mother to meet you. I want you to know that I will never come and get this baby or change my mind. I see myself as the surrogate. I wanted to meet your happy and smiling faces and tell you this baby is for you."

Doris, Bob, the girl's mother and the attorney all burst out in tears. The girl consoled her mother and when her mother finally stopped crying long enough, she told everybody that the tears were really "tears of joy."

"She said we were all blessed," Doris said.

At the time, however, no one realized how blessed. David was born in October 1986. He was immediately brought home, where Bob was in a cast and recovering from his latest surgery. Doris and Bob fed their blue-eyed blond baby—a gurgling little infant—while cradling him in Bob's most recent cast. "He fit the cast perfectly," Bob said. Bob and Doris didn't work for the first year of David's life so that they could bond with the greatest gift they had ever received. They were so in love with this boy.

Five years later, Doris was helping David dress one morning when she noticed his glands were swollen. She took him to his pediatrician, who found nothing wrong. Doris' inner voice told her to persist. She took him several times again to the pediatrician. Then she called her friends in the medical field. His blood count was fine, X rays were clear. Doris took him to several other doctors and finally went to an infectious-disease specialist who suggested David's glands needed to be biopsied.

Then the pediatrician called later and asked Doris: "Have there been any other symptoms you can think of, anything else, besides the swollen glands?"

"Night sweats," Doris said. "He has night sweats."

That's when "hell began."

The tests finally revealed that David had a rare form of non-Hodgkin's lymphoma. A tumor was later discovered in his stomach. David wound up with Dr. Jerry Finklestein, a medical director at the Jonathan Jacques Children's Cancer Center at Long Beach Memorial Hospital.

Finklestein sat David and his parents down and told him they were going on a long journey. The journey would be up the largest mountain David had ever seen, and it would be a rough journey, one with many peaks and valleys. No matter what, the doctor told David, you must always vision yourself on the top of that mountain—

at the very, very top—and never let go of that vision.

The next six months, David went in and out of the hospital having intense chemotherapy. He was put on some of the most toxic drugs imaginable. Doris quit reading the possible side effects of the drugs—blindness, deafness, nausea—because she was afraid she would stop the process out of fear. David went bald. He lost his eyebrows and his eyelashes. He had seven blood transfusions that he was told carried "magic" because the blood was all donated by friends and family.

It was clear David never thought for a second he would die. After all, look at his dad. His dad had cancer. He was still here. David felt like getting cancer was normal, like getting a cold, the measles or the chicken pox. He thought that he had something just like his dad and that he would be fine. Doris and Bob never talked to him once about death. They believed they must show a united and strong front. They never showed David how scared they were.

They moved in to the hospital and slept on the floor of David's room each time he went there, sometimes as long as 20 days at a time. The first time David went in for chemotherapy, Bob lay on the floor sweating, reliving his own experience and knowing full well what his son was going through.

When David threw up from the chemotherapy, David's parents explained that his body was driving out the bad cells that were hurting him. And once again, the school came through. Cards poured in. People made food for the family. Everybody rooted for David.

All that was three years ago. David is now nine. He goes to school regularly and has not shown a spot of cancer in his body for three years. Recently, he was so compassionate and understanding about illness, even at his young age, that he wrote a loving letter to his mother's friend who was diagnosed with breast cancer.

Dear Winnie:

I had cancer too. You are going to lose your hair, but it will grow back. Do not be afraid. If you get a headache, put your fingers on your temples, rub them forward one time and go backwards. That will help it for a minute. The medicine makes you go to sleep. Don't concentrate on the thought of the needle. Just look the other way. You will be better soon. Listen to your doctors, for they will give you instructions that you'll understand. Say "FIGHT THOSE BAD CELLS. FIGHT THOSE BAD CELLS." You'll be strong later. Don't worry. You may throw up. That is the bad cells and all the medicine getting out of your body. Tell your husband and your daughters and son that they should give you breakfast in bed, lunch in bed and dinner in bed and watch a lot of TV. You are in my thoughts.

Love,
David, Age 9

Doris and Bob know that had it been a 17-year-old mother or perhaps just any mother who hadn't dealt with cancer before, the swollen glands probably would have been missed and the cancer would have raced through David's body like wildfire. To this day, they believe that because of the magical way David came to them, he was meant to come to them—simply so they could save his life.

While David battled his illness, his parents won a trip to Mammoth Lakes.

When he was better two years later, they climbed Mammoth Mountain. There the three of them stood together, looking toward the sky. They had made it to the top.

Diana L. Chapman

An Affair to Remember

It is a curious thing in human experience but to live through a period of stress and sorrow with another person creates a bond which nothing seems able to break.

Eleanor Roosevelt

We met in January of 1995. Although I was 54 years old and he was young enough to be my son, we were to spend many hours together under the most intimate circumstances.

His room was cold and sparse with one huge bed that was hard as a rock, but with a lovely skylight that changed colors as the photo equipment he used circled the room. He often left me alone in the room, but I knew he was always close and watching me from his vantage point. This is not the beginning of a love story but the tale of young Dr. Wollman, my radiologist.

After breast surgery he became my best friend. On our first visit he informed me that seven weeks of fun was about to begin. He explained in layman's terms what to expect and showed me the room and the equipment that would be used to radiate my left breast. The first visit is the longest, at least 45 minutes of immobility while the machine is set and the target spots are put on your body—my first and last tattoo, by the way. After the first two weeks of radiation, which was five days a week for a grand total of four minutes a day, the radiated area takes on a look of intense sunburn. Not only that, but the breast that is being treated goes from a size B cup to a size C or better. Wearing a bra is out of the question and the heat that radiates from the treatment area is unbelievable.

It is amazing the thoughts that go through your mind while looking at the skylight and waiting for the treatment to be over. One comes to know the caregivers as well as their families. My Dr. Wollman and his staff were there to boost my morale whenever they thought I was down. I think I even boosted theirs from time to time. They might not have known it, but the hug they gave me whenever I walked in for treatment made it worth the discomfort and panic that I experienced each time.

During those seven weeks, I prayed, told jokes and meditated. When the time came to "graduate," as we call it, I cried as I bid my new family good-bye. However, I still see the dear doctor, and there is always that big smile and the warm hug that lit up my life for seven weeks. I shall never forget these caregivers and hope that every cancer patient that needs to go through radiation/chemotherapy is as lucky as I am. One is fearful at first because of the unknown; however, with the right attitude and doctor, it can almost be a cherished memory.

I had my first mammogram in October and everything is fine. It is important that we as women know our own bodies and if in doubt with one diagnosis, get a second or third if necessary. Had my new doctor not insisted that the small cyst come out, I would have ignored it. I will continue to live life to the fullest and be here the same time next year and the years after that. After all, there are many sunsets to watch and much love to give. My hope is that for all of you there is a Dr. Wollman and your affair can be one to remember with fondness and no regrets.

Linda Mitchell

Simply Hold a Hand

If we doctors would admit our mortality, then we would find a way to succeed with even the sickest of our patients, sometimes simply holding their hands when they are frightened and in pain, other times helping them understand the meaning of their illness and how they can use it to experience life and love. It is my patients, out of their kindness and their wisdom, who have taught me this, and it seems to me that whenever I am in danger of forgetting it, another patient helps me return to that knowledge.

Bernie S. Siegel, M.D.

You've Got a Friend

When you're down and troubled
And you need some loving care
And nothing, nothing is going right

Close your eyes and think of me
And soon I will be there
To brighten up even your darkest nights

You just call out my name
And you know wherever I am
I'll come running to see you again

Winter, Spring, Summer or Fall
All you have to do is call
And I'll be there
You've got a friend

If the sky above you
Grows dark and full of clouds
And the old north wind begins to blow

Keep your head together
And call my name out loud
Soon you'll hear me knocking at your door

You just call out my name
Winter, Spring, Summer or Fall
All you have to do is call
And I'll be there
You've got a friend

Ain't it good to know
You've got a friend
When people can be so cold

They'll hurt you, and desert you
And take your soul if you let them
O, but don't you let them

You just call out my name
Winter, Spring, Summer or Fall
All you have to do is call
And I'll be there
You've got a friend

Carole King

Dear Dr. Terebelo

It is this intangible thing, love, love in many forms, which enters into every therapeutic relationship. It is an element of which the physician may be the carrier, the vessel. And it is an element which binds and heals, which comforts and restores, which works what we have to call—for now—miracles.

Dr. Karl Menninger

May 28, 1992

Dear Dr. Terebelo,

I'm tempted to say I want to thank you now that it's over, but I know it's not. I know that for the next year, while most of me is laughing and enjoying, a part of me will hold back and watch from the shadows and pray. But enough!

I chose you as my physician because I heard you were good and that's what I was looking for. I wanted someone who really knew his stuff, would give me the facts, be a clinician and leave me alone. I was tough. I could handle anything. Thank you for knowing your stuff, being a clinician—and not leaving me alone.

Thank you for trying to educate me. When I was told I had cancer, I felt as though I had suddenly lost control over my own life. (Perhaps because I had?) The only way I could even begin to cope was to learn. Thank you for letting me have access to everything, for being honest and for teaching me—or at least trying!

Thank you for saying I wasn't a wimp, for helping me realize that there is a difference between resting and quitting.

I'd like to say thanks for the medicine, but I'm not quite that masochistic. What I will say is thanks for all the time you spent helping me deal with the medicine. I was always amazed that every time I was in your office, you never seemed rushed. Even when I behaved like a brat, you sat patiently and listened. Thank you for giving so freely of your time.

Thank you for understanding the tears. I tried to tell myself it was okay to cry, but I hated the tears. I was just so scared. Never have I felt so frightened, frustrated or helpless. Thanks for letting me cry and still hold onto my dignity. (I still regret not having stock in Kleenex.)

Thanks for all the pats and handshakes—touch can be healing, too.

Thanks for trying to teach me patience. (I think it may be a lost cause.)

And, no matter what the future holds, thanks so much for doing your best, for knowing that, especially when I'm scared, I need to be involved. Thanks for arguing with me when it really mattered. (Those closest to me think you are quite brave.)

Love,
Paula

P.S. Something that finally dawned on me is that there isn't an answer to every question or a cure for every disease. I never expected you to cure me. Quite simply, I did not hold you responsible for the results of the treatment. But I expected you to do your best. By doing that, you gained my trust. By caring, you gained my respect.

Paula (Bachleda) Koskey

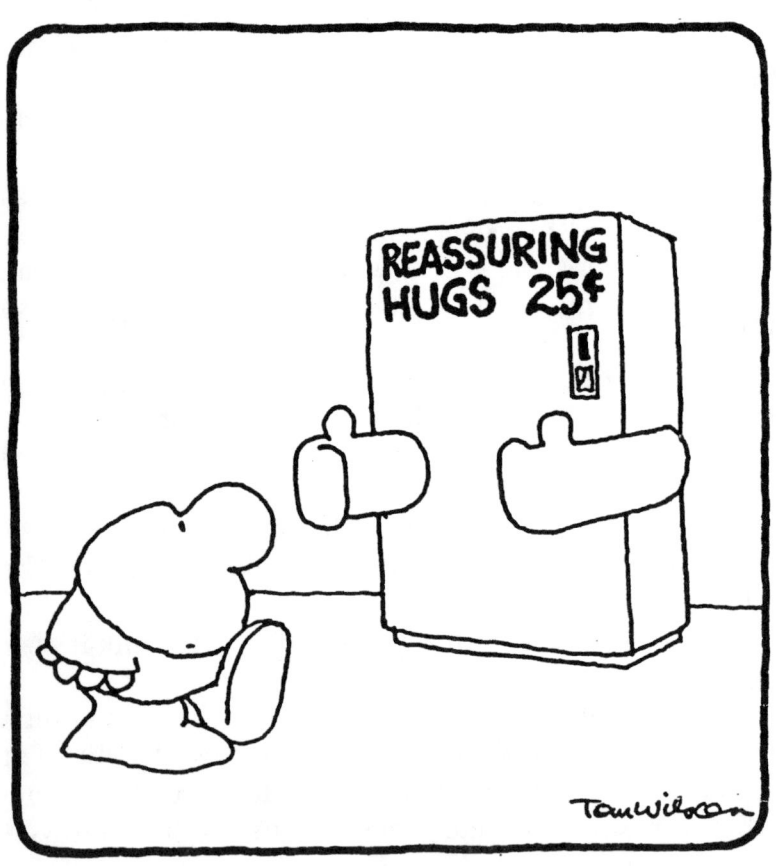

Ziggy ©Ziggy and Friends. Distributed by Universal Press Syndicate. Reprinted with permission. All rights reserved.

To the Nurses of the World

You evangelists of encouragement, you are so much
more than you know.
You have never let what you couldn't do stop you from
doing all you could do.
You are sales people, your briefcases are filled with a
product called hope.
You are explorers, knowing that once you have gone as
far as you can see, you will see farther.
You are singers spreading the melody of consideration.
You are lawyers making a case for life.
You are authors helping others add more pages to their
books of memory.
You are comedians dispensing the medicine of laughter.
You are artists who paint pictures of health on the
canvas of imagination.
You are magicians creating real miracles that inspire
patients and families.
Like King Arthur and Joan of Arc, you are warriors
battling against the villains of negativity.
Dorothy would have reached Oz much faster
In the company of one nurse—for no one can

Practice your profession unless they already possess
A brain brimming with wisdom, boundless courage, and
   a heart filled with love.
You are living proof that humanity is created in the
   image and likeness of God, and the name of that God
   is Love.

John Wayne Schlatter

The Healing

The moment hung suspended. Dr. Nathan hesitated, looking down at some papers in front of him. I waited, my senses almost painfully heightened, intensely aware of the blue-and-white pattern of his tie, the hissing radiator in the corner and the muffled sound of New York traffic outside. He looked up, and before he could speak, I read the bad news in his eyes. *Oh, no, don't say it, don't say it,* begged an inner voice. But he did.

It was very hard for him, I could tell. His kindly face couldn't hide his distress. Three years earlier he had fought and stemmed the cancer in my body, removing my left breast and then rejoicing in every year of health that followed. Now he told me that the new tumor, swelling out like an evil egg between my ribs, just below the collarbone, was "inoperable."

"We'll start cobalt right away," he said quietly. "The most important thing is not to give up."

But I already had. I knew what inoperable meant. It meant death. The trip home to our house on Manhattan's 19th Street was a numb blur. As I prepared dinner, watching my husband, Scott, and my little daughter, Erika,

playing a game at the kitchen table, a terrible anguish separated me from them like a great invisible wall. I turned
toward the stove to hide my tears.

We sat down to our meal together. The lamplight shone
warmly on Erika's face, outlining the wisps of blonde hair
that escaped from her braids. She raised a forkful of peas
to her lips, took a sip of milk, a bite of bread. Very soon, I
thought, these things that I've always taken for granted
will be lost. Erika eating, drinking, smiling, moving her
hand—all will be lost, all lost to me forever. She lifted the
fork again, and suddenly I found myself gazing at her in
astonishment.

Something had changed. I saw Erika and the world
around us differently. My daughter's simple acts of eating
glowed like precious jewels, her every movement filled
with magic and beauty. My inner eye opened to the radi-
ance of every movement. To the mystery of a Presence—
creative in everything—in the slightest gesture of her
hand, in the little green peas on her fork and in my joy at
witnessing them.

Surely, I almost said out loud, this was the work of God,
for I felt myself alive forever in the heart of the present,
alive in the very heart of Him Who caused my own to beat.

I reached for the balm of that moment, that special
awareness of being alive that God gave me, again and
again during the weeks following. But I found it increasingly difficult to recall the experience and to get in touch
with its meaning. The cobalt treatment induced deep
fatigue and nausea. Fighting the disease sapped me completely of energy. I'm tall, five-feet nine inches, and my
healthy weight is 140 pounds. By the end of the treatment
the cancer had eaten me down to 95 pounds. Now we
would have to wait and see if the treatment had an effect.

Scott, too, looked more and more drawn as he tried to
cope with household chores, his demanding job in public

relations and the fear he kept inside. One Saturday, while I napped, he dialed the Boston phone number of our dear friend Sheila. She had a deep knowledge of many subjects and read widely, keeping up with all the latest advances in the world of medicine.

Scott poured out his despair to our old friend. "I can't bear just to stand by and watch while Sybil wastes away," he told her. "I feel so helpless. Can you think of something else we could do now that she's completed the medical treatment? Something that might build Sybil up?"

Sheila understood. "There's someone I think you should call," she said.

When I awoke, Scott was sitting by my bed. I could tell that he was excited.

"I've just been talking on the phone to Sheila," he said. "She told me about a woman who helped her cousin recover from cancer. She's a scientist and professor of medicine named June Goodfield. She's British, but she lives in Michigan part of the time and she's there now. Sheila gave me her number. She's a Fellow of the Royal Society of Medicine and she's devoted years of her life to the study of cancer. Sheila says she's been all over the world doing research and interviewing patients and scientists. She knows every approach that's been tried."

Scott's excitement was contagious. "Let's call her right now," I said.

"I already did, I couldn't wait," Scott answered. "Let me tell you about it and then if you want to, we can call her again." He took my hand. "You're going to think some of this is strange, but listen for a minute, okay?"

I nodded.

"I talked with her about your case, and she asked a lot of very good questions. We were on the phone for nearly an hour. She said what you need—immediately—is a total change of scene. She told me to take you and Erika out of

New York right away and go out West. To someplace quiet and beautiful."

"What?" I was astonished. "Why?"

"Because in her experience, a drastic change in environment can trigger a change for the better. That's what happened to Sheila's cousin. Dr. Goodfield said to call the cousin and talk to her about it."

Scott seemed to have already made up his mind, but I was full of doubts. It all seemed too weird. Too quick. What if this woman was some kind of a quack? But no, she was, after all, a member of the Royal Society of Medicine, with an international reputation.

"What about your job?" I said, voicing another doubt. "And what about Erika's school? We can't leave just like that."

"Darling, that's what I thought too, at first. But Dr. Goodfield says the quick change to a totally different environment is an important first step."

"Do you believe it?" I asked.

"Somehow it makes sense to me." Scott said. "It worked for someone we know and can talk to. And besides," he squeezed my hand, "I want us to try everything that has even the smallest chance of turning you around. We have everything to lose by not trying. And we have everything to gain by going—we've tried everything else."

Three days later Erika, Scott and I got off a plane at Santa Barbara Municipal Airport and stood in the warm California wind. "We're going to put some weight on you so you won't blow out to sea," Scott said, smiling. I leaned against his arm and fought back tears. I still found it hard to believe the depth of support I was receiving. Scott's boss assured him his job would be waiting; friends and family rallied with financial help to add to our meager savings.

"I feel like a horse everyone is betting on," I said to Scott, trying to lighten the moment.

In the tranquillity of a cabin on the beach, with the clean sound of the waves and a loving atmosphere of hope and trust, I gave myself body and soul to the task of reinforcing the cobalt treatment by opening myself up to serenity in my life. In New York I'd been reading material by authors like Lawrence LeShan, Carl Simonton and Erik Peper, who described using classic techniques of relaxation, self-awareness and meditation to overcome illness. Now I used these techniques in an effort to draw as close to God as humanly possible.

Six times a day I lay down on my bed for 15-minute sessions of deep meditation and prayer. On my back, breathing deeply and regularly, I brought all of my attention to focus on the inhalation and exhalation of my lungs, on the life-giving oxygen that united me to all of God's nature on this earth. When I felt very calm, I went on to an even deeper relaxation, telling my toes to give up their tension, then my ankles, calves and so on, up my body. By the time I reached the crown of my head, I was vividly aware of my body as a living being, conscious of the blood streaming through my veins, of the warmth of my hands, feeling God's will in the beating of my heart.

Now I was ready to begin visualizing my tumor's destruction. Already I had carefully studied photos of malignant tumors, had looked long and hard at magnified portraits of the killer cancer cells and their enemies, the white blood cells. I wanted to see my target accurately.

With closed eyes, I focused my mind on the tumor like a laser beam. I "watched" as my white blood cells, wave after wave of mighty warriors, attacked and destroyed the tumor, holding the image clearly and strongly.

Finally I called up a picture of myself glowing from head to foot with vitality and health.

Day after day in our peaceful retreat, with the blue Pacific to rest my eyes on and its lulling sound constantly in my ears, I waged my campaign. Prayer. Deep relaxation. Meditation. Seeking special moments when I could see God and feel His presence in the most commonplace events, as I had seen Erika at the dinner table that night in New York.

A week went by. Two. No change. One day I sat with Erika at the table while she worked at writing the alphabet in cursive script, something she found difficult. Suddenly she threw down her pencil and burst into tears. "I'll never be able to do this, I just can't." Frustrated, she laid her head down on the writing tablet.

I stroked her hair. "I know how discouraged you feel. Sometimes things need a lot of practice and patience to work. Then all at once—bang—you've got what you've been working so hard for. Have faith and you'll see. You'll do it."

The words rang in my ears. I realized I needed to hear them myself.

On the morning of the 20th day, after 120 meditation sessions, I woke up and stretched. The cabin was still. The curtains stirred at the window and tawny California sunshine streamed in. As usual, my hand crept to my shoulder to touch the familiar, evil lump bulging out from between my ribs. My fingers stopped and spread out. Where is it? My palm rested on smooth, flat skin. I sat up and swung my legs out of bed. Slowly, almost tiptoeing, I walked to the mirror. I took my hand away. It's gone! The horror was truly gone. The tumor was completely absorbed. There was no evidence it had ever existed.

"Scott, wake up! Erika, come quick!"

Weeping, laughing and thanking God, the three of us burst out onto the early-morning beach, hugging each other and dancing with joy. Then Erika knelt and picked up a smooth white stone. "Here, Mommy, this is for you," she said as she slipped it into my hand, "so you can remember this day forever."

Twelve healthy years later, I still can't say whether the cobalt alone would have healed my tumor. I have kept the little stone that Erika gave me. Its very ordinariness reminds me that, though human problems are as plentiful as pebbles on the beach, faith in God gives us a singular power to overcome them.

Sybil Taylor

Kindest Cut

It was a bold and bald-faced—or rather, bald-headed—act of friendship: On March 11, 13 fifth-grade boys lined up to have their pates shaved at the Men's Room, a San Marcos, Calif., hair salon. Valuing substance over style, the boys embraced the full-sheared look because their classmate Ian O'Gorman, 11, about to undergo chemotherapy for cancer, would soon lose his hair. Says Ian's pal Erik Holzhauer, also 11: "You know, Ian's a really nice kid. We shaved our heads because we didn't want him to feel left out."

If compassion were a subject, the Bald Eagles, as the boys now call themselves, would clearly get A's. They took notice in early February that Ian was starting to lose weight. Then on February 18, doctors removed a tumor the size of an orange from Ian's small intestine. The diagnosis was non-Hodgkin's lymphoma, which has a 68 percent survival rate after five years for children under the age of 15. Two days later, Ian's best friend, Taylor Herber, came to the hospital. "At first I said I would shave my head as a joke, but then I decided to really do it," says Taylor. "I thought it would be less traumatizing for Ian."

At school he told the other boys what he was planning, and they jumped on the *baldwagon*.

"Soon," says Erik, "just about everyone wanted to shave their heads." That included a few girls, who never went through with it, much to Erik's relief—"I don't think Ian wanted to be followed around by a bunch of bald girls," he observes—and Jim Alter, 50, their teacher, who did. "They did all this by themselves," he says. "They're just really good kids. It was their *own* idea. The parents have been very supportive."

Ian, who completes his chemo in May, is already well enough to be playing first base on his Little League baseball team. "What my friends did really made me feel stronger. It helped me get through all of this," he says gratefully. "I was really amazed that they would do something like this for me."

And they won't stop until it's over. "When Ian gets his next CAT scan," vows Erik, "if they decide to do more chemotherapy, we'll shave our heads for another nine weeks."

People Magazine

Taking Time for Tenderness

I jerked on my seat belt and backed the car out of the garage, oblivious to the signs of early spring that usually gladdened my heart. I was on my way to my friend Joan's birthday breakfast, but I felt tight as a coiled spring. My mother-in-law, Penny, had come to live with us after a series of heart problems and small strokes. And since her arrival it seemed I'd done nothing but care for her.

This morning I'd maneuvered Penny to the edge of her bed, sponged soapy water over her body, rubbed lotion into her wrinkled skin, and brushed and braided her long hair. And as I did it, I wondered: How could she just sit there and say nothing, with me working so hard? If only she'd give me one word of thanks for the total, daily care I gave her. All she said as I put scrambled eggs and whole-wheat toast in front of her was, "I wish I could have something sweet. With cinnamon and sugar."

"Sugar's not good for you, Penny," I said, fighting to keep the tension out of my voice as I settled her in a chair by the phone and started out the door.

It wasn't fair. Penny's helplessness threatened to crowd out my simplest daily pleasures. I didn't even have time to take a break for a cup of tea, to enjoy the springtime. A dozen times a day I found myself wondering, *What about me?*

I blinked back tears as I parked the car and hurried into the restaurant. There sat my friend Joan. Her husband, Butch, had Alzheimer's disease and she devoted herself to his care. I couldn't imagine how she kept going year after year.

"Happy birthday!" I exclaimed as Joan greeted me with a hug. When I sat down, I discovered a package at my place, wrapped in tissue paper and tied with silver ribbon.

"Joan, what's going on? It's your birthday."

"Just open it," she urged.

Inside was a beautiful oak wall plaque. "Blessed be the God . . . ," read the gilded inscription, "who comforts us in all our affliction so that we may be able to comfort . . ." (II Corinthians 1:3-4, New American Standard).

"Joan, it's a treasure," I whispered, awed by a friend who gave presents on her own birthday.

"I thought you could hang it where you can read it often," she said. "I discovered that verse one day, and it changed me as a caregiver."

"So that we may be able to comfort." Words quite a bit different, I thought, from "What about me?"

Joan pushed back wisps of gray hair. "When Butch got sick," she said, "all I could think of was myself. I was so tired, so guilty, so angry. But each day God always found ways to comfort me—in the touch of a friend's hand, in the beauty of the seasons, in the smallest ways. And in the same ways that God comforted me, I started searching for ways to comfort Butch."

"Like what?"

She laughed. "Nothing big there, either. It turned out the littlest things made him happiest, too. Like reading the comics to him, even though he doesn't understand much. Or putting a ribbon on the cat. Or popping corn and watching the news together."

I thought of Penny back home in her too-quiet room. Had I been so caught up in caring for her body that I forgot her spirit? For the first time, I tried to think of what might bring joy to her day instead of mine.

After Joan and I said good-bye, I drove to the grocery store. Near the entrance were pots of bright spring flowers, and I selected one bursting with tulips. Then I headed for the bakery, then home.

"Mary?" Penny called as I opened the door. Her hands were folded in her lap on the newspaper exactly as they'd been two hours before.

Impulsively I planted a kiss on the top of her head. "I need to take a break, Penny," I said. "How would you like to have a cup of tea together? And an apple Danish?"

Her eyes lit up. "With cinnamon . . . and sugar?"

"With cinnamon, and sugar. And fresh tulips!"

"It would be wonderful. Oh, Mary . . ."

"Yes, Penny?"

"Thank you," she said.

Mary Vaughn Armstrong

Practical Tips to Help the Seriously Ill

- Don't avoid me. Be the friend . . . the loved one you've always been.
- Touch me. A simple squeeze of my hand can tell me you still care.
- Call me to tell me you're bringing my favorite dish and what time you are coming. Bring food in disposable containers, so I don't have to worry about returns.
- Take care of my children for me. I need a little time to be alone with my loved one. My children may also need a little vacation from my illness.
- Weep with me when I weep. Laugh with me when I laugh. Don't be afraid to share this with me.
- Take me out for a pleasure trip, but know my limitations.
- Call for my shopping list and make a special delivery to my home.
- Call me before you visit, but don't be afraid to visit. I need you. I am lonely.

- Help me celebrate holidays (and life) by decorating my hospital room or home, or bring me tiny gifts of flowers or other natural treasures.
- Help my family. I am sick, but they may be suffering, too. Offer to come stay with me to give my loved ones a break. Invite them out. Take them places.
- Be creative. Bring me a book of thoughts, taped music, a poster for my wall, cookies to share with my family and friends. . . .
- Let's talk about it. Maybe I need to talk about my illness. Find out by asking me: "Do you feel like talking about it?"
- Don't always feel we have to talk. We can sit silently together.
- Can you take my children or me somewhere? I may need transportation to a treatment, to the store, to the doctor.
- Help me feel good about my looks. Tell me I look good, considering my illness.
- Please include me in decision-making. I've been robbed of so many things. Please don't deny me a chance to make decisions in my family or in my life.
- Talk to me about the future. Tomorrow, next week, next year. Hope is so important to me.
- Bring me a positive attitude. It's catching!
- What's in the news? Magazines, photos, newspapers, verbal reports keep me from feeling the world is passing me by.
- Could you help me with some cleaning? During my illness, my family and I still face dirty clothes, dirty dishes and a dirty house.

- Water my flowers.
- Just send a card to say, "I care."
- Pray for me and share your faith with me.
- Tell me what you'd like to do for me and, when I agree, please do it!
- Tell me about support groups like Make Today Count (MTC), so I can share with others.

Saint Anthony's Health Center

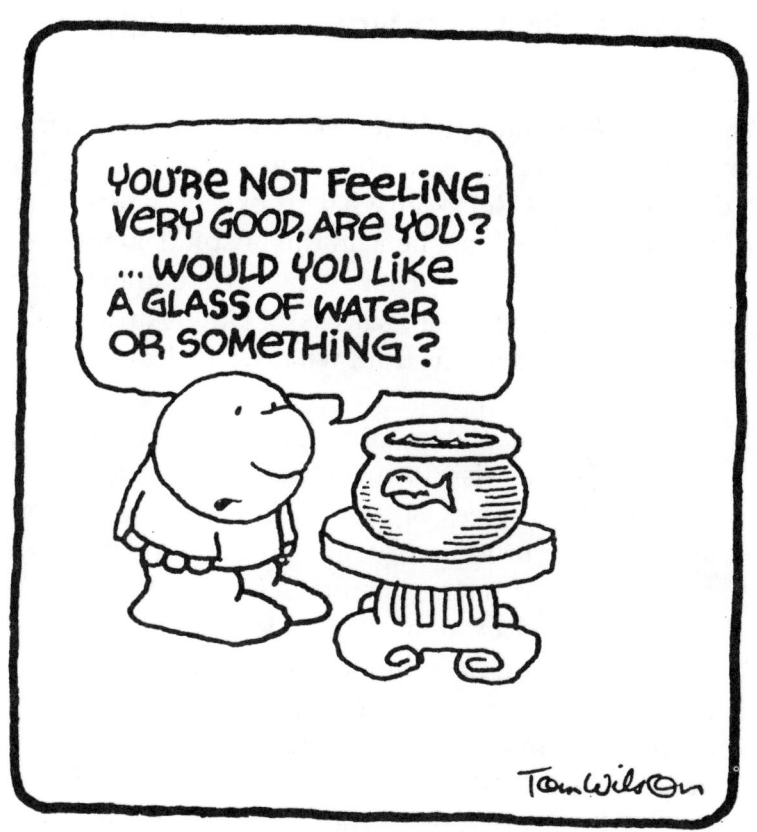

How to Make a Sick Child Smile

Our 11-year-old daughter, Rebekah, is hospitalized frequently for treatments. Beforehand, we always talk with the doctor and tell Rebekah what to expect, addressing her fears. But then when she is in the hospital, loneliness and boredom often set in. That's when we're grateful for all the friends and relatives who ask, "How can I help?" Here are a few suggestions from what we've learned.

1. Visit. Visitors are an important part of the healing process. Young visitors, especially, help children in the hospital feel less isolated. Rebekah always perks up when her brother, Bryant, comes by. If you have a young friend in the hospital, check the rules and take your children along. Talk quietly if the patient is asleep. Don't discuss the negative details of the disease in front of the child. If a doctor is present, wait for the examination to be finished, then visit.
2. Send cards. Mail notes and cards to the child's home—the parent will check the mail. Let your youngster create a homemade card or draw a picture. Once, Rebekah's Sunday school class made a

banner and a giant card with a special message from each classmate. Rebekah was thrilled and displayed them in her hospital room.

3. Bring gifts. The best kind are ones that can be shared. One friend brought a new game to the hospital, but instead of handing the gift to Rebekah, she played the game with her. Rebekah's grandmother brought a coloring book and they spent the afternoon coloring together. Don't bring candy or snacks without checking with the parent first. Gifts that stimulate the mind, such as crayons, books, puzzles or tape cassettes, are always appreciated.

4. Spend the night. If you're a close relative or friend, consider sharing the responsibility of spending a night at the hospital. It is important for those in constant contact with the child to take a break. My husband, Nolan, and I alternate. Nolan tells funny stories and I read books, but Rebekah often enjoys the comfort of a different familiar face.

    One evening when Rebekah was especially tense, my friend Donnette, a first-grade teacher, insisted on spending the night at the hospital. She always seems to cheer my daughter up. That night the two of them stayed up late, talking and giggling, relieving much of Rebekah's anxiety.

5. Entertain. Despite hectic routines, hospitalization can be very boring. How grateful I have been for celebrations organized by the hospital staff. When the circus was in town, they arranged a costume party for the children. Rebekah was a princess, and it didn't seem to bother her that she had an I.V. attached to her arm.

    If you know someone in the hospital, think imaginatively. Can a few members of your church choir drop by for some singing (and not just at Christmas time)? Do you have a friend who can perform magic tricks or dress as a clown? How about taking a birthday party to the hospital? Don't wait for the patient's birth date—do it now.

6. Pray. "Don't be weary in prayer; keep at it; watch for God's answers and remember to be thankful when they come" (Colossians 4:2, The Living Bible). Send a note that simply says, "We are praying for you." Notify the church when a child is hospitalized. Rebekah has been comforted to know that our pastor and staff prayed specifically for her.

With a little thought and creativity, you can make a sick child's day brighter. Let the child know that you are aware of the illness, care deeply and are praying daily for a recovery.

Marilyn Phillips

The Way Back

Her medical chart said that she was in her mid-30s, but framed by the four white corners of an overstuffed pillow and the high collar of a lacy pink bedjacket, her small face looked more like that of a lost and frightened little girl.

"Mind if I open the blinds?" I asked.

"Whatever," she responded listlessly.

I pulled the slender cord and the tiny hospital room was filled with the gray, wet light of a rainy day.

"My name is Doris Knight," I smiled, pulling up a chair. "Your doctor suggested that I stop by for a visit."

Still, she stared straight ahead.

"You see," I continued, "eight years ago, I had breast cancer, too, and the same kind of operation that you just had. Your doctor thought we might talk about it."

"I'd rather not," she said in a low voice. And then, slowly, she turned to face me, eyes filled with fear and desperation. For a moment, I became lost in their bleak and empty blueness. Looking beyond her, my mind spun back to a cold and drizzly Sunday morning in October, 1970. . . .

Nestled in an easy chair by our warm and crackling fireplace, I tried to find the strength to tackle an endless list of long-overdue thank-you notes. I'd been home from the hospital for three weeks, but it was the first time I'd been left alone.

My husband, John, was at church. Our 27-year-old son, Steve, was a continent away, stationed at San Diego's U.S. Naval Air Station. My sister, who flew in from out-of-state to be with me, had returned home to her family yesterday. And two days had passed since I'd heard from any of my friends—loyal neighbors, church members and coworkers. Loneliness, until now held at bay, swiftly enveloped me.

Equally disheartening was my extreme discomfort, weakness and inability to do the simplest chores. Just getting into and out of my clothes was a task of staggering proportions. Back zippers and hooks were impossible. I spent the entire morning getting dressed.

And I was depressed. Gone now were the blessed sedatives and painkillers that had made life bearable for the past few weeks. And gone with them was the spunky trouper, the incredibly cheerful optimist whose post-operative good humor had elicited choruses of "Gosh, isn't she wonderful" from friends and family. In her place was a 53-year-old scared and hurting woman.

How I longed for someone to talk to. Lurking in the darkest part of my soul were deep-seated fears too painful, too horrifying, for me to even admit. I knew I needed more than the expert medical counsel provided by my doctors. I needed more than the well-intentioned pep talks proffered by my friends. I even needed more than the unspoken love and compassion that showed in the eyes of my husband. What I needed was someone to talk to—a woman, perhaps, who had been through this whole ugly ordeal herself and who could understand firsthand what I was going through.

Reaching for a pen, I brushed against the corner of a slim volume of inspirational verse, a gift from a friend, that had been balanced on the arm of the chair. It clattered to the floor. Without thinking, I bent to pick it up. I moved too quickly. Searing pain, like nothing I'd ever felt before, pierced my chest.

"Why?" I sobbed. "Why?"

All the fears I had been trying to repress were unleashed at once with savage fury. A barrage of words, nightmarish and taunting, swirled behind my closed eyes. Breast cancer . . . malignancy . . . mastectomy . . . prosthesis . . .

I shuddered and pulled my robe more tightly around me, trying not to notice my oddly concave right side. I knew the pain was temporary; that the jolt I had just suffered was merely damaged nerve endings in the slow process of mending. I knew that with time and exercise I'd be able to resume near-normal use of my affected side. The doctors had said so. But the ugly scar would be with me forever.

Where, I wondered, was God? How could He have let this happen to me?

Never had I felt so helpless. I was especially worried about my career. After working for the telephone company for nearly half my life, a few months ago I had finally found my niche as staff editor for one of the company's statewide magazines. It was rewarding, challenging and exciting work. But it was also a job that required strength, stamina—and self-confidence. I felt no longer qualified.

More than anything else, I was worried about my husband. John, who had been a tower of strength, had a severe health problem of his own. A victim of worsening emphysema, he soon faced early retirement and needed me more than ever. In those fast-approaching days, how would I, a crippled half-shell of a woman, ever be able to give him the love and support—emotional and physical—that he deserved?

If only I had someone to talk to. Surely other women who survived breast cancer had suffered similar problems.

I wondered how they coped. I wondered what they knew that I didn't.

Again, I reached down to pick up the fallen book. This time I moved slowly, deliberately, bending from the waist. The book had landed face-up. Picking it up, my eyes were drawn to two short lines of verse.

"This body is my house—it is not I.
Triumphant in this faith, I live and die."

The author was unknown, but the words seemed to have been written expressly for me. I reread the passage out loud. It had a strangely calming and soothing effect.

With this in mind, I resolved to stop worrying—at least for the moment—and concentrate all my energy on getting better. After all, I reasoned, I should be thankful. I had survived.

Settling back in the deep, soft chair, I closed my eyes. Listening to the falling rain, the crackle and pop of burning embers, the steady, rhythmic ticking of the old clock in the hall, I slept.

Two months later, I was strong enough to return to my job. I worked hard. Most evenings I came home too exhausted to worry about anything more complicated than slipping into something loose and comfortable, fixing a simple supper for John and myself, and going to bed.

As time went on, the ragged scar healed, leveled out, and all but disappeared. I was fitted with a standard prosthesis and, to the casual observer, my appearance was absolutely normal. Still, a part of me died inside whenever I saw the curious eyes of those who knew about my operation travel to my chest. It was even worse when encountering someone who was obviously doing everything humanly possible not to look. It wasn't until some time later that I realized what a wide variety of highly sophisticated, natural-looking breast forms were available. I splurged on one of the more expensive ones. It was worth it. Before long, I was comfortable and confident wearing it all day long, and my self-image improved considerably.

It would be misleading to imply that every day thereafter was sunshine and roses. There were bad moments— undressing before a mirror with a too-critical eye, or waking in terror in the middle of the night when dark panic threatened like a storm cloud and unreasonable fears swept through me like a cold wind. John, however, was always there to hold me close and whisper words of reassurance and encouragement.

One spring day, I received a letter from the American Cancer Society. "Mrs. Knight," it read, "your name is on our list as having recently undergone a mastectomy. Would you be interested in helping to organize a local Reach to Recovery* chapter in your community for women who have undergone similar surgery?"

Through enclosed brochures, I learned that the Reach to Recovery program was founded in 1953 by Mrs. Terese Lasser, herself a mastectomy patient, and today has active chapters nationwide. The program depends on trained volunteers, all former mastectomy patients, who call new patients and help them adjust to their various psychological, physical and cosmetic needs.

The planning meeting was scheduled to take place at Valdosta's Mental Health Office, 7:00 P.M., on a Wednesday night. Aching and tired from a full day at the office, I almost didn't attend.

---

* You can contact Reach to Recovery by writing to Reach to Recovery, c/o American Cancer Society, 1599 Clifton Road North East, Atlanta, GA 30329, or by calling 800-ACS-2345.

It was a good thing I did. It was an evening of discoveries—most notably that my struggle with cancer had left me not handicapped, not less of a person, but uniquely qualified for a highly specialized service.

My gaze returned from the hospital window to the despondent young woman lying on the bed. Her breakfast tray, I noticed, was untouched.

"I understand how you feel," I said softly. "Would it be all right if I just sat with you for a while?"

"If you like." She looked away and busied herself folding and refolding a green cloth napkin.

"I'm just so darn weak," she murmured. "I can't find the strength to do anything."

"Yes, I know."

"And I'm so sore, it hurts me to even move. Especially my elbow—here, where I've been leaning on it."

Ah, I thought. Just the break I'd been waiting for. I reached in my bag for a doughnut-shaped piece of foam rubber.

"Here," I said, "rest your elbow in this."

Accepting the soft cushion gratefully, she smiled. For the first time since our meeting, the veil of fear that clouded her pretty blue eyes lifted.

"I really do understand how you're feeling," I repeated. "But there's no reason why, with time and effort, you can't be just as useful, productive, whole and happy a person as you were before your operation. I know how unbelievable that may sound at the moment, but it's true. And that's why I want you to feel free to talk."

From then on, our visit was easy. Question followed question, and soon we were engaged in lively conversation. Together we worked on the prescribed simple therapeutic exercises. She followed with interest as I walked my fingers up the wall and grinned ironically when I told her we referred to that one as "Climbing the Wall." Before we knew it, 45 minutes had flown by and it was time for me to leave.

"Now remember," I said, playfully wagging my finger. "Next time we meet, I want to hear you've been climbing the walls!"

She actually laughed out loud.

And in that sound was sheer joy and relief—for both of us. Her laughter seemed to travel back in time to soothe my own pain of eight years ago when I, like she, had so desperately needed someone to talk to. In a sudden flash of insight, I better understood the wonder of God's working in our lives; how He, in His own time and ultimate wisdom, can use the most hopeless and tragic human conditions for eventual good.

It had stopped raining, and yellow sunlight streamed in through the open blinds. As I gathered my bag and coat, I couldn't help but smile. I couldn't recall when I'd ever been happier.

Doris Knight

Reach to Recovery

In 1979, I was a 37-year-old single mother of an 11-year-old girl and an 8-year-old boy. I was an executive secretary for the president of an office systems company. As I dressed for work one morning, I hooked my bra in the front, moved it around and my left hand brushed under my left breast, detecting a lump.

I was unaware of breast cancer; there was none in my family or among my acquaintances. Perhaps because my father had passed away six months earlier from lymphoma, I immediately contacted my gynecologist. Neither he nor the surgeon he referred me to was suspicious of cancer, but suggested a biopsy. We were all very surprised when indeed the lump was malignant. In 1979, a modified radical mastectomy was my only option, and within four days I had the surgery.

While in the hospital, I was visited by a volunteer from the American Cancer Society's Reach to Recovery program. She walked in and said, "Hi, I'm from Reach to Recovery and I've had the same surgery you just had." I can't express the feeling of hope and relief I had just seeing how lovely, healthy and happy she looked! I knew at that time that I wanted to participate in that program someday.

I can't say for certain why I bounced back so quickly, but I know the tremendous support from family and friends was a huge part of it. I often wonder if the bone-deep pain I experienced—was still experiencing—with the end of an 11-year marriage could have actually helped; cancer seemed to pale compared with the imminent divorce. But the necessary attention to my lovely children and helping my incredible mother recover from the recent loss of my father encouraged me to recover from the surgery and rebuild my life.

Two years later I became reacquainted with my first boyfriend, who had moved to Nevada when we were in high school. We had a long-distance telephone relationship for a few weeks, during which he mentioned a proposed visit. But I had not told him about the mastectomy. His mother had died of ovarian cancer, and I wasn't sure how he would feel. I figured I'd better tell him, and he would never have to make the trip.

So I just said, "By the way, one thing I failed to tell you was that I had breast cancer and a mastectomy a couple of years ago."

There was a silence on the phone. Then I heard, "How about your teeth—any bridgework I should know about?" Ross and I were married six months later on a friend's ranch in rural Nevada.

We discussed the possibility of a recurrence so were somewhat prepared 18 months later when I discovered a lump in my remaining breast. I was offered a lumpectomy but opted for another mastectomy for many reasons including cosmetic—now I could be any size I wanted! Again I was blessed with no positive nodes and an easy recovery. I must admit I was pretty angry this time. I'd been taking good care of myself, I was very happy, and my life seemed to be going well. Luckily, I had lots of activities and involvement to keep me busy. I also had taken over the Reach to Recovery program in Reno, which helped my own recovery.

I've enjoyed 14 years as a Reach to Recovery volunteer, unit coordinator, and currently Nevada division coordinator. It is so satisfying to visit newly diagnosed breast cancer patients and provide a positive picture for them! Although I did not choose to have reconstructive surgery, I am aware of how important this procedure is to some. I was pleased to testify before the Nevada Legislature in 1983 in support of a pending bill that mandated that insurance companies that cover mastectomies also cover reconstruction. The bill passed. I helped the National Breast Cancer Coalition and am proud of the progress that has been made in research funding as a result of its efforts. Currently I speak to groups advocating early detection—clinical exams, self-exam and mammograms. In November 1994, I participated in a city-wide campaign called "Buddy Check," which encourages women to get a buddy and remind each other to do their breast self-exam each month. It has received a positive response, and I continue to represent the program through the media and personal presentations.

Three years after my second mastectomy, I was diagnosed with acute lymphocytic leukemia and underwent 15 months of aggressive chemotherapy and radiation, which certainly got my attention! I believe I experienced every emotion and side effect possible—a real roller coaster: Not a hair on my body for over a year, unbelievable weakness and fatigue, nausea and mouth sores, emotional highs and lows—but definitely more good days than bad; more "ups" than "downs." I think the successful experiences with breast cancer set me up for expecting good results, and I am pleased to be in my ninth year of remission! The three cancer experiences inspired me to return to college and get a degree in Human Development and Family Studies—a B.S. at 50! Now I am on call for cancer patients at a large medical center that involves me with the patients and their families. I also co-facilitate a weekly cancer support group in the hospital, provide personal consultations, and coordinate the "I Can Cope" program for the American Cancer Society. I feel very strongly that cancer patients need to see people who have "been there" and offer survivors, family members and those in treatment an opportunity to explore all the ideas, tools, theories, resources—whatever it takes to heal.

I am so thankful that I am here to enjoy life with a husband who has not let me down for a minute throughout the past 14 years. I was thrilled to be here to see both of my children graduate from college and to plan my daughter's June 1995 wedding! My son just got engaged and will be married next summer. My cancer experiences taught my children that cancer need not be a death sentence, and they also learned some things about facing adversity and winning. It is tough to ever be depressed, as I feel life has been very good to me.

What advice would I give someone facing the cancer challenge? Everyone is so different and each situation so unique, I can only say what works for me:

1. Have a genuine and close partnership with your physician(s) that includes getting as much information and education as you wish;
2. Trust that whatever therapy (chemo, radiation or both) will work;
3. Let your body dictate your level of activity—don't push; on "good" days, do something fun and/or meaningful;
4. Visualize yourself healthy, strong and vital, and bring up this image in your mind several times a

day and before you go to sleep;

5. Allow people to do things for you—it is the best gift you can give them at a time when they feel helpless;

6. Make a list of all the things you want to do and places you want to see before you die and review it regularly;

7. Get in touch with whatever spirituality is meaningful to you and make it a partner for healing;

8. Keep that cliché, "positive attitude," as much as possible, but don't become its prisoner—it's okay (and normal) to have some bad days, to cry and scream, "It's not fair!" Trust that these feelings will pass;

9. Join a support group and try coping mechanisms and stress reduction techniques that others suggest. Then continue dropping in on the group after recovery to offer inspiration for others;

10. Slow down and appreciate the wondrous details and miracles happening from moment to moment.

I think I love the work I do because of the incredible inspiration I am privileged to encounter every day with cancer patients. There is an aura of courage and strength that permeates the oncology unit and continues throughout the support group. I feel it in telephone conversations as well as in the warm hugs patients, families and friends exchange regularly—as if somehow the strength and love are highly contagious and healing. Would I recommend that everyone get a little dose of cancer in order to feel this way? *Heavens, no!* I do believe, however, that my life would not be as precious and meaningful had the cancer experience not happened to me.

Sally deLipkau

Taking Charge

I was a 57-year-old real estate developer in 1984 when I was diagnosed with late-stage lymphoma, cancer of the lymphatic system. My doctor told me my chances of recovery were slim. I remember that I spent the days immediately following the diagnosis talking about suicide. I often burst into tears. I had given up and I was sure I was going to die soon. Although I had family and friends, I felt alone. I wouldn't let them be with me. They couldn't understand—they didn't have cancer. They weren't doomed to die.

But Marsha, my wife, urged me to try The Wellness Community. Although I was depressed and could hardly walk, and was still sure I was going to die, I went. I met all kinds of people who were fighting for recovery who didn't seem nearly as depressed as I was. I joined a group, started doing direct visualization, changed my diet, began learning about cancer, took back control of many areas of my life, and started acting like a human being again . . . and wonderful things started happening. The crying spells vanished. I started enjoying life for the first time in many months, and my physical condition started improving.

Today, almost 12 years later, I am still without symptoms. Up until two years ago, I was back at work full-time. Now I'm retired, but still take good care of myself. I am absolutely convinced that my participation in my fight for recovery played an invaluable role in that recovery. I don't believe I would have survived if I had not received wonderful medical treatment, and if I had not taken the actions I did to help myself get well. Without either, I was a goner.

Phil

A Special Mission

Little did I dream in April of 1986 how much a "cluster of microcalcifications" could alter my life. Whether it was God's will, bad luck, the fates or a strong genetic predisposition (my mother, two aunts and sister have also coped with breast cancer), my life was greatly affected by that first diagnosis.

I am Sister Sue Tracy, O.P. (Order of Preachers), a 55-year-old Polish-American, Grand Rapids Dominican Sister. Detroit is my original home, but my 36 convent years have provided me with many "homes" along the way. Ministries have included junior- and senior-high teaching, vocation directing for my religious congregation, parish ministry throughout northern Michigan, and now hospital chaplaincy. Since 1989, I have served as pastoral care director at Mercy Hospital in Toledo—much more a joy than a job.

A special focus of my hospital ministry has been contact with other persons coping with cancer as well as their families. Interacting with so many resilient people has been one of the beautiful side effects of cancer. On my 50th birthday in 1990, I became an American Cancer Society Cansurmount volunteer and added the Lucas County Unit to my "homes"—truly a place of comfort and challenge.

In January 1993 cancer revisited. Three things emerged: (1) I wanted God to be glorified come what may; (2) I wanted to learn the life lessons inherent in this breast cancer recurrence; and (3) I wanted to remain in charge, networking with the doctors not as a victim but as a partner. I felt very much responsible for my part in the healing process.

My American Cancer Society contacts have been a vital part of the holistic healing experience since May of 1986. Reach to Recovery was the first contact that enhanced my shaky hope; I Can Cope served as a powerful means of lessening my dreadful fear of chemotherapy; Look Good . . . Feel Better was a two-hour gift of joyful connecting with other women as we all left toting a gold mine of free makeup. This year in June, I had the privilege of sharing *My Cancer Herstory* at the American Cancer Society state headquarters in Dublin, Ohio. For the past eight years, the American Cancer Society has been a valued companion in my cancer journey.

No, I would not have freely chosen cancer a first or second time. However, today I proclaim I would not trade all I have learned, lived, laughed and loved because of it. I do not consider myself just a cancer survivor with genuine respect for that commonly used term. I see myself as a cancer thriver. My basic attitude is gratitude. I know there is no guarantee this won't happen again, but I don't live just holding my breath. I treasure life. With a careful diet, moderate exercise, positive attitude and daily prayer, I keep trucking along. I believe God has bestowed a special mission to be present and supportive of fellow travelers on the cancer journey. So midst the ups, downs and in-betweens, I feel richly blessed.

Sister Sue Tracy, O.P.

7

ON INSIGHTS AND LESSONS

Life is a succession of lessons which must be lived to be understood.

Ralph Waldo Emerson

Lessons Cancer Taught Me

What an experience having cancer is. My whole life will be different for as long as I live. And, yes, I am one of those who wants to live to be a hundred. An exceptional nurse at the hospital told me to "live each day to the max." Do you know what the max turned out to be? Once I was up and around again after two surgeries in five weeks time. It was hanging up laundry in the sun with a cat rubbing against my leg.

Caryn Summers, R.N.

I am a habitually busy single woman, which is why I customarily deferred health-related matters until they reached the "crisis" stage. So it was after several months that I consulted an internist to examine a swollen gland under my ear that persisted rather than dissolved with time. After his examination, the doctor suggested that I not "bother it" if it didn't bother me. I took his advice explicitly, and he treated me for other minor complaints over a three-year period. One day I called him for a referral to a dermatologist. My hands and feet had been itching for several weeks. My doctor then suggested that I come into his office, and he conceded that he would refer me to a dermatologist if he indeed could not treat me for the itching. On that visit, I reminded him of my persistently swollen gland. He seemed shocked that he had not heard about it before. I then suggested that he check his notes from my first visit three years prior. There it was! And several weeks later, I was in surgery to have a malignant parotid gland removed. Other tumors were discovered in my chest and in back of my nose. My diagnosis was lymphoma. My prognosis was a 40 percent chance of surviving five years.

My first reaction was confusion. I wondered, "What am I to do now?" I pondered the choices. I could brood, as I've seen so many people do. I could be resentful with people around me, be angry at God, be alienated and isolated in my dilemma—I've seen that too. I've heard about some fatalistic reactions where patients decided they had to "die with something," and went along passively to their demise. There were many other ways I considered responding; but I made what I call the "interactive" choice. I chose to participate in the decisions affecting the remainder of my life—however long that may be. It was a good decision!

I began reading and learning about my illness. I read about the survival rate of cancer patients who fit my demographic profile. I read about clinical trials in experimental treatment for my disease. I read about the variety of chemical therapies that had been used to treat my disease, and the side effects associated with them. I consulted a nurse who treated cancer patients and who worked with oncologists. I read everything the American Cancer Society had in print about my disease. In the two weeks that elapsed between surgery and my first radiation treatment, I was ready to make informed choices about my treatment. The first lesson I learned is: Make informed choices. Difficult times are much easier to endure when they result from one's own choice.

Before every decision was final, I asked, "What are the options?" and then, "What are the consequences of those options?" The doctors were exasperated—at first, but eventually they expected me to have the last word. Each choice I made was a difficult one. For example, I could have waited another year with no treatment and hoped that the surgery removed it all. I could have completed a program of radiation therapy and hoped that the radiation would dissolve all the tumors. Or I could have radiation and several courses of chemotherapy, and added to that a bone marrow harvest (if and when the cancer was arrested). I chose the comprehensive treatment (radiation, chemotherapy and bone marrow harvest—in addition to the surgery). I have not regretted it. The second lesson cancer taught me is: Don't avoid hard choices. We're tougher than we think.

In my readings, I discovered the books and video-tapes of Dr. Bernie Siegel. He founded the nationally renowned Exceptional Cancer Patients (ECaP) group. He discovered that his patients who survive months and years past their prognosis are the ones who participated in the treatment decision-making! In his book *Love, Medicine & Miracles,* Dr. Siegel poses a very powerful question: What will this disease permit you to do that you did not have the courage to do before? Before my illness, I did not have the courage to say no. I was tired, but I pushed myself. I didn't believe in the things I was doing, but I did them anyway for other people's approval. The things I wanted to do for myself, I deferred because I preferred the approval of people I considered more significant than myself. Cancer changed all that. It allowed me to say no. Cancer excused me to do things I had wanted to do for a long time: rest . . . lay up and read . . . let people come to me . . . put myself first! The third lesson cancer taught me is: Love myself more. It was the love I'd been longing for.

I must be forthright with the next lesson. Look for good anywhere and you'll find good everywhere. At the beginning of my treatment, I enrolled in a Dale Carnegie Public Speaking and Human Relations course. Each person in the course was required to choose one principle to practice for the entire course. The principle I chose was: Don't criticize, condemn or complain. Immediately, I began seeing good wherever I looked for good. On the nights when pain orbited my body like an invisible satellite and I hadn't slept for what seemed like days, I was enveloped in an aura of unsurpassed peace and confidence. I learned to experience more deeply the meaning of grace.

In mid-October, my hair came out. Since the weather was too cold to go bald, I had to find a head covering that suited my wardrobe and my personality. I chose baseball caps. Actually, I now have a wide variety of them; but my favorite was fuchsia! I wore it everywhere. And now that my hair is back, I still wear it. People would look at me then and laugh, but that—at least to me—was preferable to having them look at me in pity. What was the principle of this lesson? Enjoy the humor in my circumstances! It helped other people find courage in my attitude.

Next, I decided to live more vigorously. One of the dreams I had completely abandoned was finishing college. I acquired a student loan, re-enrolled in school full-time while working full-time, and missed only one class in 14 months. On February 11, 1993, I completed a B.A. in Management and Communications at Concordia University in Wisconsin, graduating summa cum laude, and delivering the valedictory address for my class. After an eight-month rest, I enrolled in graduate school and in another year, completed an M.A. in Gerontology (with a 4.4 GPA). We can do all things through the power of Christ (which I believe to be God residing in us)! Surviving cancer actually empowered me to believe I could do *anything* else!

Over the last four years, I have volunteered as a CanSurmount counselor—mainly to stay in touch with the power of what cancer taught me. Although my cancer experience seems to benefit and inspire many people, I am enriched and empowered talking with people who are just beginning cancer treatment. On February 11, 1994—the third anniversary of my remission—I received a call at work from the CanSurmount director. She wanted to know if I would counsel another patient with my diagnosis—Jacqueline Kennedy Onassis. I consented and listened in shock as she instructed me in how to make contact with Mrs. Onassis. My next lesson was crystal clear: We are all one. In the grand scheme of things, our least common denominator is the will to thrive.

This year during National Cancer Survivor's Day, I celebrated four-and-a-half years of remission by sharing the lessons I learned from cancer with other celebrants. I think one of my most important points was this: Between those of us who view cancer as a challenge and those of us who view cancer as a curse, the primary distinction is whether we perceive ourselves as victors or victims. As a cancer survivor, I proclaim the most important lessons of my life have been taught by cancer—a severe teacher. It has taught me the best way to live: Make informed choices. Do not avoid the hard choices. Love myself more. Look for good anywhere and find good everywhere. Enjoy the humor in my circumstances. Live vigorously and remember that we are all one!

Were I to reduce all my lessons to one concise moral, I would use the letters: G-O-D-I-S-N-O-W-H-E-R-E. It can be read, "God is nowhere!" or "God is now here!" Like everything in my life of any significance, the way I see it always depends on how I look at it.

Bernadette C. Randle

No Less a Starfish

About eight weeks after my first mastectomy, I agreed to accompany my husband on a business trip to Connecticut and Rhode Island during June, with the understanding that I could rest as much as necessary and not overdo it. In an attempt to make sure we balanced pleasure with business meetings, my husband asked if there was anything special I wanted to do while we were in that beautiful part of the country. Because I grew up in Arizona with desert and dryness I have always had a genuine love of and appreciation for the ocean. I suggested we try to get down to Newport beach if at all possible. For me, there is something therapeutic about the ocean. The waves, walking in the sand, watching the tide, just experiencing the presence of the ocean. Somehow I felt I would feel more connected to nature, myself and the healing process.

Armed with a map and directions from the lady who sold us our box lunches, we were on our way. The drive was beautiful and far shorter than we expected.

We gathered our things and headed for the shore. I couldn't wait to take off my sandals and scrunch my toes in the wet sand. As we topped a hill, the beach looked like a patchwork quilt of beach blankets. I had never seen so many people on so little sand in all my life. We weaved our way through the crowd toward the water. As I took a step, I looked down, and to my utter surprise, saw a beautiful starfish. I thought to myself, *How could this be?* All those people, and no one stepped on it or even bent over to pick it up. I was as thrilled as a child. For me it was magic: my own personal gift from the sea. Then I realized something unique about this particular starfish. It had a message—a very special message. One of its arms was bent and curved around. At that moment, from someplace deep within me, I had an overwhelming awareness, a sense of meaning. This was no less a starfish because it had a bent arm, and I was no less a woman because I lost my breasts. I called it my "grace moment." I realized it was no accident that I found myself on *that* beach, *that* day, at *that* moment.

This experience was simply an answer to my prayer. I knew I would survive breast cancer from that moment on. Furthermore, I had a message I would willingly share with others.

No matter what our setbacks, difficulties or pain, we can get through them. Only through these moments of hell do we reach deep down within our being and discover who we are, what we believe and what is important and "real" in our lives. We experience a "knowing of our soul."

Today, I have my little starfish on a special table in my home. Every time I pass it I think of its message. I'm grateful for the insight having cancer gave to me and for a relationship with a Higher Power that blesses me with little miracles on a daily basis. Most of all, I am grateful to know in my heart that I am no less a woman because I lost my breasts to cancer. I am more than my limitations.

Katherine Stephens Gallagher

A True Learning Experience

On an overcast summer day, I sat on my duffel bag, sleeping bag and pillow waiting for my ride. I was filled with excitement and undue nervousness, unsure of what the next nine days had in store for me. I was on the road to volunteering for my first time at Camp Ronald McDonald for Good Times, a camp for cancer patients, ages 7 to 18. Having no idea that this would be the most amazing week of my life, I faced perplexing questions: What if I have a camper who has an emergency? What if I get an uncontrollable cabin? What if I can't handle the incredible emotional experience?

I was relieved when I was paired with a wonderful co-counselor who had been to camp twice before. Mary Anne and I instantly meshed. Pre-camp orientation ended and it was now time to head down the hill to pick up the children. As we approached the Children's Hospital of Los Angeles, my butterflies fluttered uncontrollably. One of the veteran counselors must have sensed my anxiety because he wrapped his arms around me to give me a bear hug and a simple wink to rekindle my confidence.

I decided to jump in and start having fun with these

children, who had traveled from everywhere between San Diego to Bakersfield to forget about their troubles and enjoy a week of fun. Some campers were getting reacquainted with friends from past summers. Others stayed close in the comfort of their families, in an awkward position of not really wanting to hang out with Mom, but not convinced that branching out needed to take place right then.

As I surveyed the scene, I saw a few children who were amputees, some in wheelchairs, and a sprinkling of bald heads hidden under hats or scarves, but most of the campers looked as healthy as any other children their age. I noticed there was a group of seasoned campers singing camp songs in a circle. Since this was my first year, I was not too familiar with the proper lyrics and hand motions of "Super Lizard." With a football in hand, I proceeded over to an "I'm too cool for Super Lizard" group of guys. I said, "Hi, I'm Lisa. Would you want to throw the football around?" In all honesty, I didn't know a thing about setting up a football game, but I guess I sounded convincing because before long everyone wore wide smiles. The campers were having fun, and I sensed that a week would be much too short for this frolic. I was in paradise. I was having as much fun as the campers and enjoyed meeting all the patients, all the while recruiting more players. It did not take long for this group to assimilate. The boys showed off for the girls, while the gals either displayed their athleticism or were happy just checking out the male campers. One girl told me that she already knew she wanted to ask Michael to the dance, which, keep in mind, was days away.

We loaded the bus and I knew that this week was going to be great. At camp, we were assigned our cabins. Cabin Four consisted of eight 11- to 13-year-old girls, Mary Anne and myself. We stuck together like glue through all the exciting activities during the week. We had 10 different personalities and not all were angels. However, there was something strangely wonderful about being confined to a very small living space, which contained only two small mirrors and campers who woke up at 6 A.M. to be the first to use the showers.

One night during Cabin Nine's teepee overnight, a night where each cabin gets a turn to eat and sleep outdoors in one large teepee, I was returning from taking Misty to receive her nighttime meds. We had just settled back into the warmth of our sleeping bags and it wasn't five minutes before the "C-word" was brought up. I sat there quiet as a mouse, unsure what would happen next. "So what kind do you have?" They all shared and then within the same breath someone said, "So, who do you guys think is cute at camp?" They had answered their own curiosity, in addition to strengthening the bond they already shared. It was an intense few moments, but it did not take long for these campers to continue talking about important 11- through 13-year-old topics—such as boys. Yet these girls were amazingly knowledgeable, possessing more strength and wisdom than some people twice their ages. In the course of the week, I had almost forgotten they were sick. Every day they continually battled with cancer, a disease that many times we associate with adults. Cancer is a topic that most of us cannot cope with easily or lightly. These children will always be affected by this disease, yet for one week a year they live freely, surrounded by hope, inspiration, support and love, with kids just like themselves.

It was the last night of camp after the exciting dance. Energy ran high in Cabin Four. Mary Anne and I finally calmed our little dancers down enough to leave for the dining hall for a staff meeting. Two counselors patrolled the area, and we had a two-hour reprieve. We received reports that our cabin was laughing so uncontrollably that they could be heard throughout all the girls' cabins. Curious if that was really true, Mary Anne and I peeked our heads across the barren field. All we could see were faint small lights resembling a harmless, competitive game of flashlight tag coming from where else but Cabin Number Four.

Two hours later, we returned to our cabin in good spirits and exhausted. The week had taken a toll on us. As I opened the door, Rosa was screaming, "Lisa, help!" I immediately put my arm around her and tried to ask her what was wrong. She continued to cry, trying to talk through her tears. "My ear hurts so bad; I have never been in so much pain." Oh, my goodness, I had made it the whole week without any big problems. My initial horrific apprehensions were coming true. I was so scared that something serious might go wrong that I couldn't handle, something they did not teach me at the camp orientation.

Here it was 2 A.M. and ironically, it was Rosa who was crying out for help on this day. The whole week Rosa and I had connected so well, and I had so much fun setting her up with all these dates for the dance. However, today Rosa had displayed a mean streak in her and turned vicious, especially to me. I knew this was her way to continue getting my attention. She kept pushing me until I lost my patience, which is something I rarely do, and I stormed out of the cabin. She really hurt my feelings, and I was so upset that Rosa was able to get the best of me earlier.

Now, Rosa lay in my arms, crying hysterically for me to help her. I was so frightened that something would happen to her. The other girls in the cabin were so exhausted that they rolled over and continued sleeping through all this commotion, while Mary Anne and I got Rosa dressed and over to the Med Shed. I just held her tight and kept telling her it was going to be okay, reassuring myself in the process. We woke up the nurse on duty and she checked out our terrified patient. It turned out that she only had a bad earache, and I can't tell you how thankful we all were.

Often when I am consumed with trials in my life, I reflect back on those special children who possess knowledge and maturity beyond their years. I have learned from them that in comparison, my troubles are very insignificant. As a teacher who usually gives lessons daily, I feel that I was instead taught valuable lessons on the importance of life in those nine days. Those optimistic, risk-taking campers taught me the preciousness of life, illustrating that each day is a gift and to live to the fullest because no one knows what tomorrow will bring. From this incredible experience, I learned first-hand the importance of giving yourself to others and receiving much more in return than what you gave. Thank you for these important life lessons.

Lisa McKeehan

Humor Helps

I have always set personal boundaries of what is funny and what is not. I have been quoted as saying, "There are just some things you don't poke fun at." I was wrong. Laughter rises out of tragedy when you need it the most and rewards you for your courage.

Without it, it would have been impossible to imagine how these children and their families could have endured their load.

The giddiness of a moment when 15-year-old Jessica, Burlington, Vermont, with a "below the knee" amputation, was playing soccer and not only the ball, but her prosthesis sailed through the air leaving "the tall, gorgeous, humorous person I am" convulsed on the floor with laughter.

Sometimes it was a situation that cried for perspective. Ryan was treated for neuroblastoma at age three with surgery and radiation. Eleven years later, he emerged with no health problems, but there was just one little glitch. He only perspires and blushes on one side of his body. Ryan may use less deodorant than the rest of us, but his sense of humor was left intact, as is evidenced by his artwork.

Betsy of Boston, Massachusetts, speaks of optimism and humor as her "caretakers" during her bout with cancer. It put the following experience in perspective. The 17-year-old entered a treatment room to receive her radiation therapy. Several people were already there so she dropped her gown and prepared to get on with it. Upon questioning she found that the extra people in the room weren't medical students as she had assumed, but painters there to estimate the cost of repainting the room!

Worth noting is that the incident happened in 1965, and Betsy added, "I wish there had been organizations and opportunities available 24 years ago to allow me to share 'experiences' rather than 'memories.'"

Erma Bombeck

EDITOR'S NOTE: Erma Bombeck died on April 22, 1996 due to complications from a kidney transplant. Her courage and strength exemplify the spirit of this book. We mourn her passing with great sorrow.

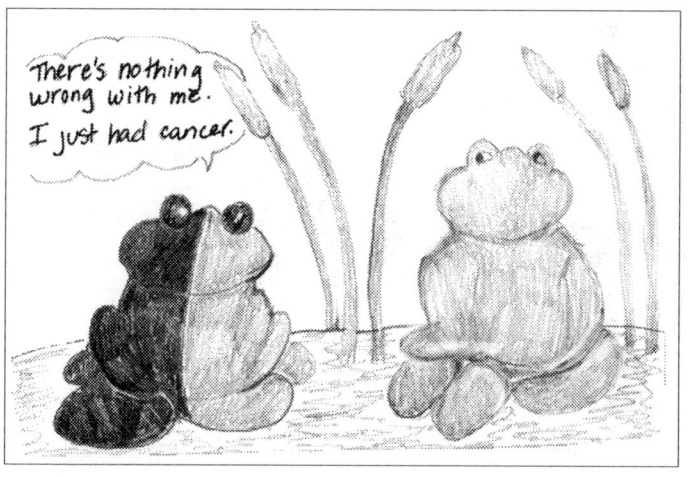

Cancer Introduced Me to Myself

One secures the gold of the spirit when he finds himself.

Claude M. Bristol

A three-day wait for the results, which I already know in my gut. Three days lying flat on the couch, staring as the television changes programs hour after hour. The phone rings. They'll cut off my breast on Monday. I am 13 weeks pregnant. I am 33 years old.

They do it. They really meant it. My right side has a 12-inch incision; no lymph glands, no breast. There are 12 more tumors in my glands.

I have three choices: immediate abortion, a cesarean section or induced labor at about 30 weeks, or a full-term delivery. My cancer is hormone-positive, and my body is lousy with hormones. I can't have any of the usual cancer therapy if I keep the baby. Even with an abortion and therapy, my chances are a shattering one in six for five more years of life.

I choose to go for 30 weeks. I don't choose it to save the baby. I choose it to get out of the hospital, so they won't do anything more to me now. They pull two long, sucking tubes out of my side, and I go home. It is January in Minnesota, as frozen as you can get, unless, of course, you are pregnant and have cancer.

When you are a human time bomb, it is a lot longer than five months from January to May. Each day my baby grows, more of the hormones, so enormously dangerous to me, flood my body. There is little reason to hope that I will complete the pregnancy with no further cancer spread. I am so numb, so angry, so very, very sad that my face freezes into an expressionless mask. I lose the ability to read (previously one of my greatest joys), because my concentration is completely destroyed. I don't expect to see my girl become eight years old on June 30, 1978. I buy all her gifts and wrap them in February. I plan my burial.

But I really was two people, each fighting hard for the upper hand. One heard what the doctors said and reacted as I have just described. But the other shouted obscenities at the hospital whenever her car passed by. This second person decided to fight, even though the first person was after her every day, sometimes every hour, to give up and give in.

Physically, my mastectomy didn't hurt very much. My chest, upper arm and back were numb, but I healed fast, without complications. But my arm hurt from the beginning, sometimes so badly that I couldn't straighten it for days. Unfortunately it was my right arm, the one I used to strum my guitar. But it really didn't matter, because I wasn't happy enough to sing anymore.

As soon as I left the hospital, I tried to listen to my insides. I wanted my body and mind to tell me how to help them survive. I got some answers, and I tried to follow them even when I was too depressed to move or care. My body said, "drink orange juice," a curious craving I'd never experienced before. I drank and drank, and it felt right. I put serious thought into what I put into my body. I told my food to make me strong. I told each vitamin, as it slid down my throat, to go to the right places and do the right things, because they were the only cancer pills I had.

My body said, "Move, Lois, and do it fast!" Thirty minutes after I came home from the hospital I went for a walk. It was hard. I was afraid of falling on my side. I was humped like an old lady. But my legs were strong. I bought a pedometer and walked off miles and miles. When spring came, I walked, ran, walked and ran, until there was too much baby.

I told my body through exercise that I loved it and wanted it to be healthy. I started yoga again the week I came home. At first I could only move my arm about five inches from my side in any direction, but I stretched and stretched it. I got my three-pound weights out and made my arm muscles and tendons work even though they protested painfully. I got my arm strength back quickly and have full mobility and strength today. Reach to Recovery says, "Walk your fingers slowly up the door." I say, "Hang on the door, and then do chin-ups if you can."

My mind and body said, "Make love," and they were right. Making love (and other forms of exercise) gave me the only times I was free, the only times I was me again, the only times I didn't have cancer.

My mind said, "I need peace. I need some rest every day from the overpowering pressure. Rest me!" I had never meditated, but I went to the library and discovered the forms that worked for me. I practiced. Meditation dropped my tense body out of my waking turmoil into a sweet cradle, deep and dark and refreshingly peaceful. I literally lived for those moments.

Meditation also provided me with a chance to practice medicine without a license. I told my body to be well. I told my immunological system to protect me. I looked at my brain, my bones, my liver, and my lungs every night. I felt them and told them to be free of cancer. I watched my blood flowing strongly. I told the wound to heal quickly and the area around it to be clean. I told my other breast to behave, because its the only one my husband and I have left. I still tell my body and mind every night, "I reject cancer. I reject cancer."

The doctors poke around, look at my X rays, let me out into the world again. I make it into spring, into May.

We try an induction the last week in May. It goes on for 10 hours, it hurts a lot, and accomplishes nothing. They, the ones not in the bed, want to try again tomorrow. Baby and I want to go home. We go, and I tell myself that three or four more weeks won't kill me! I am happy because, going full term, I can deliver with the midwives. Perhaps the birth, at least, will be beautiful even if the pregnancy was hell.

My college roommate had a baby on June 13, and I guess that I will, too. With amniotic fluid beginning to leak, I go to the hospital to a lovely room with plants and a big double bed. My midwife is good in all ways. The contractions are close and getting stronger, and I begin to lose the fear all women have. I am handling this well. I'm going to enjoy it.

She breaks the bag, and the bed and I are drenched. She says I'm six centimeters, but I watch her face change. I'm pushing the cord out before the baby. I know immediately that he could die—fast. She holds the baby's head off the cord, pushes him up as I push him down, and I now know what the word agony means. As we race to surgery, I hear them say that the baby's pulse rate is 60.

Maybe a C-section was a good idea. They spend another hour looking at my insides. They find nothing but insides, and when my husband tells me, I feel a moment of great relief.

The baby is an 8-pound, 1/2-ounce, 21-inch baby boy named Nathan Scott. He is very cute, with brown hair, long dark eyelashes—and a large ventricular septal defect, known among the lucky uninitiated as a heart murmur or hole-in-the-heart. It is congenital. It is serious. It will probably need surgery and it could be life threatening. And, worst of all for me, it means constant trips to a hospital I hate. Trips that leave me exhausted and depressed for days. It means letting my baby be cut up, just like me, for his own good.

Nathan is in danger of congestive heart failure for the first six months of his life. He takes digitalis twice a day. He sweats when he eats. His little bony chest rises and falls much too fast, and his liver and heart are enlarged. He goes into the hospital for a while. I stay with him, and it causes me nearly to break. His original 50 percent chance of closure drops to 25 percent.

But then, sometime in his seventh month, he improves. (I like to think it was during one of those moments when I was whispering in his little ear, "Nathan, you are *going* to get well!")

The doctors are surprised. The EKGs improve. He gains weight. His breathing slows and the liquid swelling leaves his liver.

In May 1979 Nate has his first normal EKG, a better event than a first birthday. The muscle has closed around the hole. Nathan pulls himself up on his feet and stands tall, and I begin to believe in his existence.

When my tummy flattened out, I had a big surprise. I really didn't have a breast on the right side. Now was the time when most new mothers love to put on their old clothes, or buy new ones, or dream of two-piece bathing suits. My tent clothes had protected me for six months. Now I had to confront my true feelings about my body, another struggle to add to all the rest.

To describe how I felt as depression is mild. But I kept pushing myself to continue the positive elements in my life. For seven months I didn't lose my baby fat, but when Nathan began to improve, I experienced a new wave of determination.

I lost 20 pounds. I continued to meditate and to swallow all my vitamins. Three months after the birth I rejoined my exercise group. Now I didn't have to walk; I could run. And I run so well I'm planning to enter some races. My exercise program consists of yoga, running and biking. I do them every day. I have to. I believe they are helping me survive.

My figure is back, with clothes on anyway. I'm even beginning to think I don't look too grotesque with them off. My C-section scar didn't do much to help my self-image, but my husband is blind when he looks at my scars, and I am learning to see through his eyes.

I began to try to learn how to put *myself* first. What I did worked, and each day of continued good health makes me more confident of "mind over matter."

I think of cancer every day, but I also think of how strong my body is, and how good it feels most of the time. I still talk to my insides. I have a feeling of integration of body, mind and, probably, spirit, which I have never before experienced. Cancer introduced me to myself, and I like who I met.

Lois Becker

Thoughts for the Year

The greatest handicap: Fear
The best day: Today
Easiest thing to do: Find a fault
Most useless asset: Pride
The greatest mistake: Giving up
Greatest stumbling block: Egotism
The greatest comfort: Work well done
Most disagreeable person: The complainer
Worst bankruptcy: Loss of enthusiasm
Greatest need: Common sense
Meanest feeling: Regret at another's success
Best gift: Forgiveness
The greatest moment: Death
Greatest knowledge: God
The greatest thing in the world: Love

Source Unknown

My Resolve
(For Today, Anyway)

August 19, 1991

This is what I've decided:

I'm tired of people telling me (and of saying) how lucky I am.

I don't feel lucky.

I know I'll survive this. I am a strong person and know my glass is half full, but please don't tell me it's full—I've sipped a few and spilled some.

I will not be beat and I will fight but I am allowed to say I'm tired. Even people who win get tired.

I've got a lot to do and plan to do as much as I can but first, if I need to cry, I'm going to do it and that's okay.

God has seen me through a lot of stuff and I know He'll give me the strength to pull this off.

I will not allow people to talk about how I can "just get a wig" and how my hair will grow back. This is a tough one for me, and I will handle it in my own way. Some issues are bigger than others, and to me, this is really a biggie.

I am going to fight—and win.

I will work at being stronger, but I won't like it!

Life is for living and complaints will be kept to a minimum. We've all got something and at least I've got people who care.

I see this thing as a sock in the stomach—it takes your breath away, leaves you sore but you end up walking away.

I will cherish life more. I am blessed with three wonderful kids and family and friends who love and care and are more than willing to help. I will learn to accept help graciously. I will learn that part of the loving act of holding hands requires that one person's hand be gently cradled inside another's. I will learn to willingly cradle my hand in those extended to me, and I will not forget to extend my hand to others.

Daily, I will pray for strength. I will not be bitter or a martyr.

I will be strong.

I will laugh.

I will cry.

I will win.

Paula (Bachleda) Koskey

My Realizations
(At This Point in Time)

May 19, 1992

When all this started, I somehow thought I would come through it a much wiser and stronger person. I don't feel as though I have. I simply feel grateful I survived. However, I cannot let such an intrusive event happen without giving it some thought. This is some of the stuff that comes to mind:

Living through one day can seem much longer than looking back on nine months. And an hour of chemo is the longest measurement of time there is.

I laugh at the naiveté of my resolve of August—and respect it. The intensity of some feelings/experiences cannot be anticipated, and a lot can be accomplished by simply holding tight.

Cancer is not like a sock in the stomach. It is a huge battle that affects every part of a person's being. I was totally ignorant of how overwhelming it can be.

I tried to make up for losing control over my life by gaining knowledge—it helped.

Sometimes ignorance is bliss.

There is such a thing as too thin. (Next I'd like to try too rich.)

I love my hair! There is something truly wonderful about rubbing my head and not having my hair fall out.

It is much better to give than to receive and much easier!

As much as it infuriated me at the time, I'm grateful to my oncologist for his single-minded determination to beat this disease.

I do have a somewhat strong will. (Why am I the only one surprised by this realization? And what do you mean—stubborn?)

Laughter, hugs and chocolate are the stuff of life!

As much as the drugs healed my body, the people who were willing to listen healed my soul.

I am still glad I never wasted time wondering why me or saying woe is me—stuff happens and is.

I am terribly in love with a whole bunch of people.

My kids are simply incredible! This battle was really tough on them, but I have a feeling that even with the scars, they will come out of this better than they were before.

I am not stoic, strong or saintly.

I am happy, huggable and hairy!

It's okay to complain about stuff as long as somewhere the good gets remembered, too.

Sometimes winning isn't what it seems. Sometimes the knowledge gained from the battle is most precious of all. And sometimes the victory is simply a deeper love of those who shared the fight.

I fought.
I laughed.
I cried.
We won.

Paula (Bachleda) Koskey

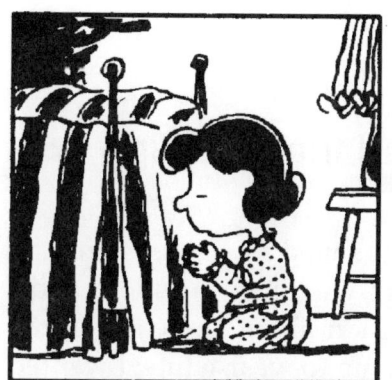
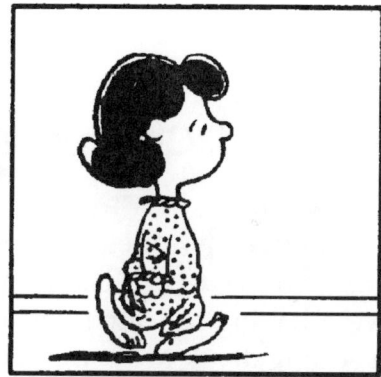
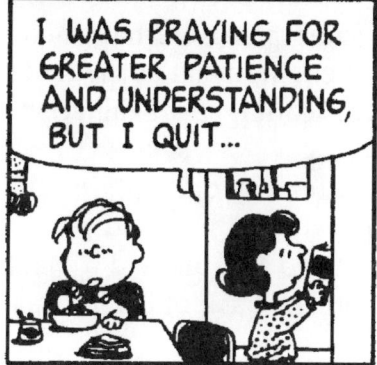
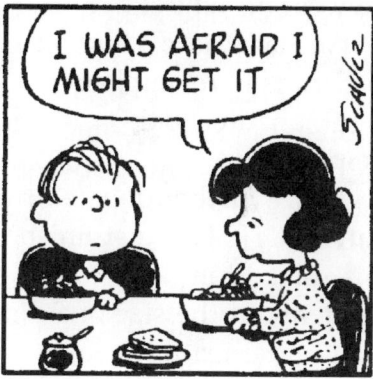

Dad, Cancer and the Wedding

An uncanny series of events saved my father's life.

About six weeks before my wedding, my mom and I were having a heated discussion about the color of my wedding dress. Mom wanted me to wear white; I wanted to wear off-white.

We had the discussion the same place we had many others as I grew up—in the kitchen. Mom sat at the table. I sat on the floor, cross-legged, leaning up against the refrigerator.

As we further debated the matter, my dad entered the kitchen. He had just finished his shower and had put on his robe. From where I sat, I noticed that he had a black spot, about the size of a dime, on the back of his left calf, just underneath the knee.

I asked Dad how long he had that dark, raised spot. He said he was aware of it, but didn't know how long it had been there. Mom said he called it his beauty mark.

I told Dad he needed to have that mark checked out. I told him about Mel, the man who used to co-anchor the evening television news with me in Michigan. His wife had noticed a black spot on the back of his shoulder. That black spot turned out to be melanoma. Skin cancer. Mel's cancer was caught in time. But, had it not been, it would have spread quickly because the spot was located very close to his lymph nodes.

Dad promised he would have his spot checked out. Mom and I continued to discuss wedding dresses.

After visiting with Mom and Dad, I flew back to Boston where I was a consumer reporter for WNAC-TV. One day after work, Dad called to tell me he had a specialist look at the spot and was sure all was okay. In fact, Dad planned to make his scheduled business trip to Boston in a couple of weeks.

The next call from my parents brought the news that Dad wouldn't be coming to Boston. That wicked beauty mark was melanoma. Doctors explained to us that there are five stages of melanoma. Dad's cancer had progressed to level three. He would need surgery to try and combat his disease.

I flew home for Dad's surgery. The doctors made every attempt to go in and scoop out the cancer. As we waited for the results to see if they were able to get all the cancer, the minutes seemed like hours, the hours like days, the days like weeks.

We knew that a level three melanoma had the potential to spread like wildfire. Not a good sign. We counted the days waiting for the results. Five days passed. The results came. His cancer was caught in time!

Dad had a hard time walking after his surgery, which took place three weeks before my wedding. He kept saying his main goal now was to be able to escort his little girl down the aisle. Dad's leg just wouldn't support his weight. At the wedding, Mom and I met Dad halfway down the aisle, where he waited for us in his wheelchair. Mom and I supported Dad as he haltingly walked between us. As we approached the altar, a friend met Dad with his wheelchair. Dad achieved his goal—he walked me down the aisle.

Since 1981 my father's body has remained cancer-free. He is checked annually. He is still vital, alive and well.

I have always remained firmly convinced that Mom and I were meant to have that heated discussion mentioned earlier. It allowed me to be positioned to see Dad's melanoma, which in turn allowed the cancer to be arrested. All of this happened because I wanted to get married in an off-white wedding gown, which, by the way, appeared white in all the pictures.

Linda Blackman

Surviving Cancer

It seems like only yesterday
my doctor told me I had cancer,
and when I asked, "How long do I have?"
he didn't have an answer.

And it seemed to me that time stood still
and the room turned upside down.
Life just stopped and I stared at him
and I didn't hear a sound.

And a thousand years flashed by my eyes
as I thought of all I'd miss,
of the laughs and smiles of those I loved
and my two-year-old daughter's kiss.

And I realized right then and there
the time that I had wasted,
of all the things I'd never done
and all the life untasted.

And I thought of all the silly things
that occupied our day,

like the stupid fight we had last night
over bills we had to pay.

Twenty years have come and gone
and I'm still at the dance.
I guess that God just changed his mind
and gave me another chance.

And on that day I took a vow
to let go of the past,
to live my life and love each day
as if it were my last.

For only God can know these things
the day, the hour, the time,
but on this day I am alive
and all the world is mine.

Jill Warren

My Story

When the call came that October evening in 1986, the voice on the other end of the phone was my obstetrician, who was also my friend.

One year earlier, she had held my hand through a very difficult pregnancy and the premature birth of my daughter, Kirtley. In fact, it was at my one-year visit just the week before that I had pointed out a small lump in my right breast, which I discovered the previous week as the result of a strange, painful itching. Neither of us was concerned. At 37 I was too young for breast cancer, and everyone knows that cancer has no feeling (two myths debunked!). But she suggested a mammogram. I sensed that it was not something to delay and went the next day.

She called on Friday night with the results. I recall her explaining that the lump would have to be taken out and biopsied and that I would have to find a surgeon. Someplace in my gut I screamed, "I can't find a surgeon, I can't do anything; I have cancer. I am going to die. I have a one-year-old daughter, and she won't even remember me." It was a thought *too* crushing to sustain for more than an instant.

I moved through the house like an image from a carnival fun house. My head went first, followed by a body that seemed to undulate from the shoulders down. My body had turned on me. It was trying to kill me.

What followed for me was five months that included surgery and chemotherapy and seven years that have included an indescribable journey into myself and out again.

Like all breast cancer patients, I'll never know the critical moment when some aberrant cell in my body decided to go haywire and begin multiplying. What I do acknowledge are factors that I believe led to my cancer. They are unique to my history and not meant to be a guideline for any other women.

But like most other women I have talked to, I needed to decide why I got breast cancer in order to better cope with it and to accept that these factors could affect my daughter's risk of breast cancer.

At 36 I became a first-time mother to a three-pound, one-ounce premature infant who didn't sleep for six hours straight until she was three months old. My diet after Kirtley's birth became more erratic at a time when I should have been building my immune system. I was emotionally and physically spent. My estrogen level had been up and down, and I was already at high risk by having had my first child after age 35.

In October 1991, almost five years to the day after my diagnosis, my mother was diagnosed, and I learned I had another high-risk factor—family history.

In addition, while information concerning birth control pills and breast cancer is contradictory at best, new studies point to those of us who took the pill in the late 1960s, when the dosage was four to five times what women take today. We took them early in our childbearing years for extended periods, and new studies (some of which are refuted by other studies) indicate that combination could result in a risk five times greater than normal for developing breast cancer.

I consider myself an open person, but the possibility that unexpressed anger was causing stress prompted me to be much more open about my feelings (my husband, Tom, says I am succeeding).

Lest I sound like one who has bought entirely the idea that I caused my cancer, I also blame our environment and the endless combinations of carcinogens to which we are exposed growing up in the 20th century. I remember clearly my pesticide-covered neighborhood—free of mosquitoes, but covered with a fine mist of chemicals twice a week. What effect, I wonder, did the twice-weekly DDT spraying have on my health? How many other carcinogens played a part in my cancer I will never know, but in spring 1992, studies showed that the breast tissue of women who had breast cancer showed much higher levels of PCBs found in pesticides! How I can protect my daughter from the possibility of breast cancer in light of all the questions for which there are no answers is another set of issues.

Physically, I have recovered well from breast cancer. After undergoing a modified radical mastectomy in October 1986, I underwent six rounds of chemotherapy due to one malignant lymph node.

The chemotherapy experience can only be described as the most difficult thing I have ever experienced.

I also know I would do it again in a minute after researching this issue for more than two years (and the introduction in 1990 of the anti-nausea drug Zofran, which has eliminated nausea for a significant percent of women). I have also talked to women who lost only part of their hair and bounced back well. It isn't easy watching your hair accumulate in the drain, but it is easier than watching your baby toddle toward you knowing you aren't doing everything possible to ensure you will be around to rear her.

In 1981 I had a back-flap breast reconstruction. My back muscle was moved to my chest wall, along with a wedge of skin, and a silicone implant was placed underneath it. The nipple was formed with skin from my upper thigh and then tattooed to match the existing nipple. The left breast was lifted to match the newly constructed breast. No, I don't look the same. I have a long scar down my back, and the scars on my reconstructed breast are still a little pink. But I can move my new breast, and I am gradually regaining feeling in the armpit and surrounding areas. And with the changes on the left breast, my chest looks like it did when I was 18: firm and straight ahead!

While I am constantly amazed at the physical result of reconstruction, I was totally unprepared for the enormous emotional change that occurred after reconstruction. In a way, I am whole again physically. When I'm dressed in bathing suits and nightgowns, no one would know I ever had breast cancer.

I wish my soul and psyche were so easily restored. Emotionally, I remain on the roller-coaster ride that is life after breast cancer. On my good days, I praise medical science for the speed and efficiency with which it removed the cancer. I think of myself as a cancer survivor and even find myself grateful for chemotherapy. I can even have a sense of humor about breast cancer from time to time, and on my good days I list the positive changes cancer wrought in my life. My panic attacks are farther apart now, and I no longer lie in bed and cry quietly as I wonder how my daughter will cope with adolescence after I have died.

On my bad days I have a pain that quickly becomes chronic. Sure that I am dying, I call my oncologist. But the bad days are fewer now than last year, which was better than the year before that. I just read one statistic that says it takes us three years to (choose one) get over, assimilate, cope with, recover from, deal with breast cancer. No, I don't think "get back to normal" is a choice in that sentence. How your life will change as a result of breast cancer is up to you.

I have learned a number of things about myself since discovering I had breast cancer. Before my diagnosis, I was in the middle of the postpartum blues as I tried to decide personal directions. I was irritated with little things. My prayer life consisted of questions such as, Where am I going? What do you want from me? Help me see what is important in life.

Now I know what is important. And while I cannot call my cancer a gift, it certainly clarified my life for me and provided a few truths:

> *I can live without a breast.*
> *Relationships are not based on breasts.*
> *I have a high pain tolerance.*
> *I don't like to vomit.*
> *Hair grows back.*
> *Children grow up no matter what.*

On a more introspective level, I have accepted that I had cancer, but that fact does not have to ruin or rule my life. I have a lot to live for, and I intend to live for it. I know now that fear can be more painful than surgery. But most of all, I know I now have the personal power to make my own decisions.

Kathy LaTour

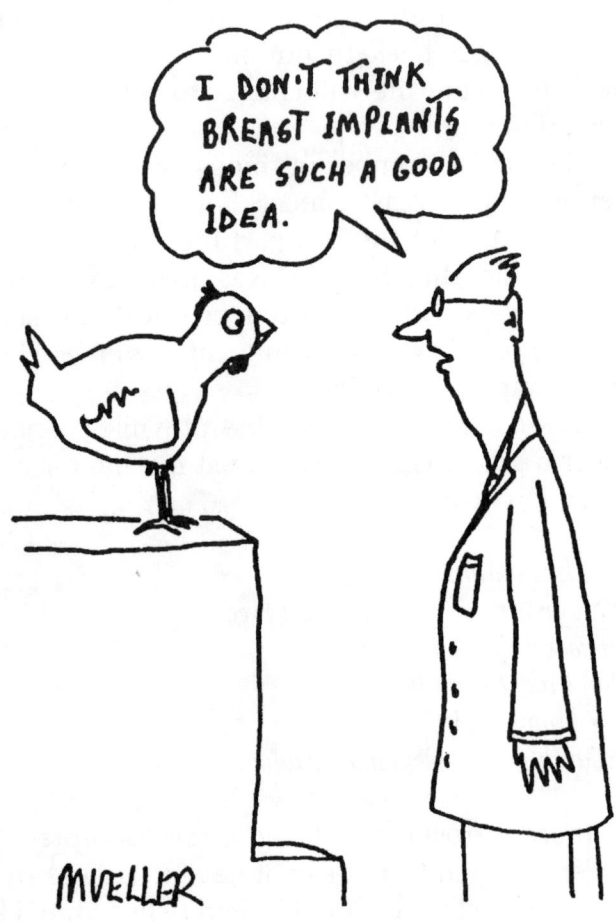

Reprinted with permission from Pete Mueller.

Live Your Life

I was severely depressed. I had helped a friend through a traumatic and dangerous situation, and all of my well-intentioned help only seemed to make matters worse. Feeling lost, I sat down on my daughter's bed in despair. My eye caught a crumpled piece of yellow paper with the attached wisdom:

> *The past is gone, but Now is Forever. The future does not lie in our hands, but the future lies in the hands of the Present. Go out and grasp the seconds of the day as if you had only that day to live. Experience and enjoy the moments of your life. We only have one life to live, so live it like a champion. Everyone was put here for a purpose, so let that purpose rise up above and show everyone what you're made of.*
>
> *I'm not telling you how you should live, but how you should feel when you look back at the memories of a once-upon life of yours. Don't regret things later. If you feel it is right, do it. It's your life and nobody else's. Make decisions that please you. Let nobody put you down. Don't live in anybody's shadows or dreams. If you do have a dream, act on it and it will probably come true.*

I was amazed by what I read; the words spoke right to my soul and brought light to my mind. I ran to my daughter and asked her where she had found this piece of writing, thinking that she must have copied it from some magazine. She shyly admitted that she had written it herself. "But you're only 12!" I exclaimed. "How could you have written this? Where did you learn this from?"

"Don't you know, Mom?" she replied. "You've taught me all this! I just wrote it all down."

Judy and Katie Griffler

THE FAMILY CIRCUS
Bil Keane

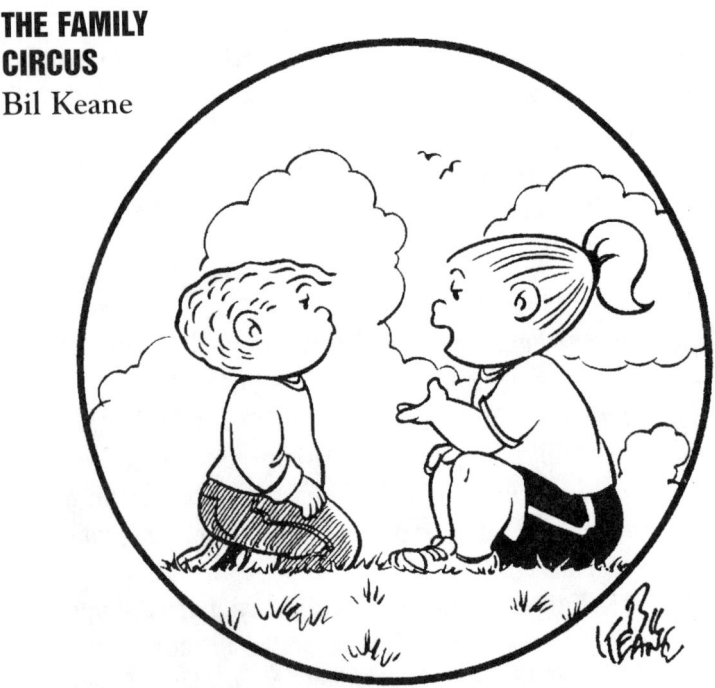

"Yesterday's the past, tomorrow's the future, but today is a GIFT. That's why it's called the present."

Twenty Minutes Is a Lifetime . . .

Diseases can be our spiritual flat tires— discrepancies in our lives that seem to be disasters at the time, but end by redirecting our lives in a meaningful way.

Bernie S. Siegel, M.D.

Fourteen years ago, I was a woman like any other. Married, mother of two children, manager of an optical shop, I led a seemingly normal existence. At 49, I had explored a variety of experiences. Between my extravagances and my traditional values, my concerns and certainties, I struggled to cope with my daughter's adolescence and my husband's absences. The common lot, I suppose.

May 1982
A routine checkup
A blurry spot in the eye
A life collapsed by a few frantic cells
A cancerous tumor, 12 millimeters in diameter
In the eye

Doctors call it malignant "melanoma"
Many examinations, only one verdict:
Inoculation or death . . .
Without appeal . . .

In an instant, I tumbled from the world of healthy
people into the world of the ill. The beatings of my heart
became the beatings in my head. When I shut my eyes, I
saw the concerned faces of doctors, my ears resounding
with their judgments. I couldn't believe that I was going
to survive. I felt as if I had been erased from life.

I was disturbed, suspecting that perhaps my illness had
deeper psychological aspects. Unconsciously, facing
death brought me back to another pain, one inherited
from a Jewish childhood invaded by Nazi occupation.
Born in 1933 in Paris (the same year Hitler came to power),
my early memories revolved around hiding, fear and
shame, hungry for food, hungry for love and having no
rights. The pain of my disease uncovered a whole series of
anguishes, the depth of which I had barely suspected.

In looking at my life prior to the diagnosis, I noticed
other points of stress and conflict. My daughter, Lara, was
having her adolescent crisis. Suddenly, I no longer had
the right hair, nor the right words—and certainly not the
right attitude. My husband's business kept him abroad,
and I felt my life unraveling around me. In this chaos, my
cancer brought unexpected responses to unfulfilled vital
needs. My daughter's crisis ended immediately and my
husband stopped traveling! Little by little, I realized that
in my life, disease had often played a crucial role, an
anchor amidst my insecurities. It enabled me to hook onto
other people, to induce their concern and make them
caress me, "tender" me, tell me "I love you."

I had been running after love all my life, and yet I
began realizing that the source of love was within me. In

my darkest moments, my family's faith was the rock I clung to. Although there was little reason for hope, they made that hope an absolute priority in our lives and never let their fears undermine it. Beneath the threat of cancer, we came together as a family, rediscovering each other as we searched a path of health. There was my son, Noah, nine years old. School did not interest him very much, but one day he was going to receive his high school diploma. That, I wanted to see! And Lara, my daughter, so radiant, so ravishing. . . .

I felt cornered by the impenetrable wall of cancer, but I realized there must be another side. More than ever, I wanted to go there.

I was simultaneously told, "You're going to die in a few months," and "Think positively." It wasn't possible for me. I was too afraid. I was unable to shift from "you're going to die" to "you're going to heal." Whenever I thought about my future, the terror overwhelmed me. I woke up every morning shaking with fear: "I'm going to die in the next 20 minutes!" Until the day I was fed up: "Okay, you are going to die in the next 20 minutes . . . *so what!?* So what are you going to do in those 20 minutes?" This "so what" got me to face the essential questions, not as an intellectual exercise but as an experience.

I also met Dr. Carl Simonton, who helped me change from "you cannot heal, you will die" to "you can die"—not "you will die," but "you can." He recentered me on my goals, not my fears. That was an extraordinary shift. I became active in my healing and stepped out of the ghetto of disease, reentering the vitality of life, finding the courage to tell myself: "I can, I can, I can. . . . "

The more I chose what I wanted for myself and others, the more a great life force stirred within me. I learned to trust the idea that "you can heal and what you do today makes a significant difference." Acting upon this belief was my first step on the path of healthy thinking—what a discovery, not just for my cancer, but for my entire life.

Feeling impelled to tell healthy people that they don't need to wait for a disease or a very serious event in order to transform their lives, my husband and I started sharing our experience and eventually founded an international institute called Au Coeur de la Communication (At the Heart of Communication). Dedicated to creating healthy communication between individuals, families and communities, this process of supporting and sharing with other people, and gradually designing educational programs, propelled me back into the world of human beings, leaving behind an atmosphere completely dominated by my cancer. This was an essential starting point for me. As I widened my vision upon others and the world, I sensed that it infused my body with vital strength and energy. I cherished more and more the present moment. Each morning found me still alive, the days turning into months. Deftly, quietly, cell by cell, my energy, the quality of my life came back.

My journey with cancer taught me to question my certainties. The most difficult part to overcome was my own unhealthy beliefs about life, death and disease.

I learned that I could make each moment essential, choosing to reenter the flow of life, abandoning an addiction, reconciling a misunderstanding, rekindling a relationship. Now, Au Coeur de la Communication explores this through programs in the fields of health, education, business and intercultural dialogue. How can we as individuals make a difference in our families, our health, our organizations and in the world?

I've rediscovered life—my "response ability" in it, for it. For all this, I can now fondly say, "My dear cancer!"

Claire Nuer

Finding My Passion

There is in the worst of fortunes the best of chances for a happy change.

Euripides

I know a lot about passion because in the process of living, I lost it, but in the process of dying, I found it again.

My life was about three things: pleasing, proving and achieving. I thought that if enough people liked me, I would feel better about being me. I wanted desperately to please everyone . . . family, bosses, neighbors, people I didn't like. It hardly mattered who they were; other people's approval and validation were the source of my self-esteem. "Looking good" was my daily regime, and I was incredibly good at it. I continually quested for greater and greater accomplishments because those proved my value to the outside world.

This thinking affected the entire fabric of my life. My work was a series of long hours, proving my dedication and making sure I never offended anyone. I made impossible promises that were hard to keep because I was afraid to say no, which added untold amounts of stress. By constantly reacting to outside circumstances rather than taking charge of my life, I felt victimized and I lived in fear that "they"—whoever "they" were—would suddenly discover I was incompetent. The fact that I was the youngest woman in my company to hold an executive position and became director of corporate communications while still in my mid-20s did not assuage my concern. Nothing soothed my self-doubt.

The only solution I knew was to try harder, work longer, achieve more. I just knew I'd be happy when I did the right thing. I left the corporate world knowing that being independent would change everything. Ironically, I became a career consultant and taught people how to look good and be aware of what others expected of them. I knew all about that.

Of course, I was still a people-pleaser and took lower fees because I feared no one would use my services. Instead of being driven by the demands of a boss, I was driven by the demands of my clients. I couldn't understand why I was financially struggling and assumed the answer was to simply make more money. So the cycle escalated as I decided to increase my marketing and promotion efforts even more. When I burned out and grew discontented with no improvement in my income, I decided there was something intrinsically wrong with me and embarked on a campaign to fix it. I went to classes, lost weight and joined personal-growth groups. I was still empty.

So it went . . . my life of pleasing, proving and achieving. What did it get me? Tired. Broke. Emotionally depleted. And terribly afraid.

Then in 1986, the awakening came. I discovered I had bladder cancer and the prognosis looked bleak because my symptoms could be traced back for three years. My doctor had the bedside manner of a blacksmith and was not gently encouraging. In my first surgery, he removed the largest tumor he had ever taken from a bladder and announced we would be doing another surgery in 10 to 12 weeks "to see what was left." This is a fun guy.

The cancer changed my life forever. I made a decision to live, and that had a number of implications. I gained immediate clarity about what was important and began focusing on becoming well. I changed my diet, discovered herbs, explored holistic healing and learned what it meant to take care of myself.

Most important, I began asking the question: Who am I and what am I doing here? Previously, my concern was: What does everyone else want and how can I make them like me? I shifted from being involved with the changing demands of the outside world to focusing on what was in my heart. This was not an easy process, since I had spent my whole life looking outside for answers. I was so accustomed to ferreting out what other people wanted from me, I had no idea who I was.

I realized that my life totally lacked passion ... that zest for living, that sense of joy, creativity and spontaneity that truly comprises life. Suddenly faced with possible death, I knew I had never really lived. In fact, there had been no "life" in my life. As a result of this awareness, passion became my reason for living. I committed myself to it wholly and completely!

No, I had no idea what it meant. I just knew that my daily purpose was to get up and do something passionate each day. I walked on the beach, discovered I love rollercoaster rides, took fun classes that wouldn't make me a "better" person and read books I had wanted to read for years. I made a list of things I wanted to do before I died (whenever that might be) and as I did them, the list just grew. Enthusiasm, excitement and fulfillment were ends in themselves. I wanted to fully experience and live every moment I had left. I could wait no longer.

I felt more positive and hopeful. It took less energy to produce better results. I allowed myself to be uncertain about how my future was going to unfold; I just continued exploring and expressing my passion on a daily basis. I now know the sheer force of this commitment produced miracles.

By now, my business was shut down, I had no money coming in and no one was interested in hiring a terminally ill patient. But some of my old clients began calling and asking if I would do career coaching in my home. Heaven knows, nothing else was happening, so I said yes, but my consulting took a new turn. I talked about the cancer and my commitment to living a passionate life; I thought they might want that, too. Indeed, many wanted to hear more, and I began conducting groups. By the end of the first year working in my living room, I discovered I had seen more people and made more money than I had any other year in my career. After all those years of working and trying so hard, it was that simple. What a revelation! I knew I had stumbled onto something that could work for anyone who embraced it.

The other major miracle is that I have been cancer-free since 1987. My doctor is stunned by my recovery. When I have my annual checkups, he always comments on how well I have healed. Apparently, there are not even any remaining indications of the surgery. Is this the result of a commitment to passion? While I cannot prove it to you, I don't doubt it. I believe passion is the strongest force in the universe and that it is a magnet for all one's good— happiness, power, joy, abundance and health. You know how exhilarating it can be to be around a group of passionate people. It produces a euphoric energy. Like running, it creates endorphins in the brain. Endorphins boost and protect the immune system. Cancer is a disease of the immune system, so why couldn't passion heal it?

For me, the process of dying brought great relevance to living. Today I bring as much life to living as possible. It has also become my livelihood. I built an organization called The Career Clinic, which has helped well over a thousand people heal their relationship with work through discovering their passions and purpose in life. Passion is not for the lucky or the talented; it is the fire waiting to be ignited in every soul.

Through cancer, I received the gift of life. Now I get to give it away by speaking and teaching, and do so with great gratitude and joy.

Mary Lyn Miller

What's It For?

As a breast cancer survivor, I'll be the first one to say that there is nothing funny about having cancer. But as a comedienne, I try to find humor in my everyday life. After my diagnosis in 1991, I began writing comedy material around my cancer experiences to help my own healing process. Six months later—between my third and fourth surgery—I began performing my "cancer comedy" for other cancer survivors to help bring some lightheartedness to a tough topic. I have expanded my presentation to include the physical and psychological benefits that we gain from laughter, the ways to find humor in our everyday lives, and many true and funny stories.

One of my favorite stories is from a friend of mine, Peggy Johnson, the 1995-96 Chairman of the Susan G. Komen Breast Cancer Foundation. I thank her and her son, Jake, for allowing me to share their experience.

> I have a card hanging in my shower with diagrams showing how to perform a breast exam. Usually I leave the card with the pictures facing the wall. One day, however, the cleaning lady left it turned outward. My

7-year-old son, Jake, saw it and asked me what it was for. Without going into much detail, I told him it was there to remind me to do something every month and to show me how to do it. Jake replied, "Mama, I can't believe you don't know how to wash your boobs."

I share this story to illustrate three points. First, it's a wonderful, true and funny story that makes us laugh. My motto is "Keep Laughing to Keep Healthy" because laughter is good for us. I truly believe the funniest stories are found in our everyday lives. Second, it's an excellent story of perception and shows how two people can be looking at the same thing and see something different. We all can choose how we look at things that happen in our own life, even a cancer diagnosis. Sometimes, we just need a little more information or tools, like humor, to look at things differently and change our perception. Third, I hope that when women are taking their showers, they'll remember this story and remember to do their breast exams because early detection is so important. For your very own free shower card, call the Susan G. Komen Breast Cancer Foundation at 1-800-IM-AWARE.

Jane Hill

The Best Thing That Ever Happened to Me

Happiness isn't about what happens to us—it's about how we perceive what happens to us. It's the knack of finding a positive for every negative, and viewing a setback as a challenge. If we can just stop wishing for what we don't have, and start enjoying what we do have, our lives can be richer, more fulfilled—and happier. The time to be happy is now.

Lynn Peters

Walk into any room where she is present and you'll spot her right away. Attractive, well-dressed, friendly, with a terrific smile—and a warmth that radiates from her soul to yours. She portrays the image of one who "has it all" as she laughs, smiles and giggles with such confidence and self-assurance that all there envy her in some small way. You really have to wonder where all that "can do" attitude comes from. If you ask, she replies, "It comes from a belief in myself—you see, I have survived."

No one would ever guess that this radiant woman

experienced a serious problem in her life. Every incident from her past has been carefully noted and filed in its appropriate slot in the time span called life. This woman is noted mostly for her way of always giving to others. Most of the time she does not even wait for the question of how; the answer is "yes" right away. She is cheerful beyond the normal tolerance of human nature. Spending just one hour with her can do as much for you as a month's vacation.

* * * * * *

As I read and ponder the above words used in an editorial to describe me, I feel a slight smile slide across my lips. My life has not always read as if you might like to trade places with me instantly. Recall my quote from above, "I have survived." The date was February 3, 1970, and at the age of 23, with three children under the age of 3, I was wheeled into surgery. They found a large tumor in the left chest wall, growing through my ribs directly over my heart and attempting to attach itself there. This needed to be removed immediately. And so it was. The result was an incision extending from the front of my chest all around to the back in order to remove three rib sections over my heart. The muscles to my left arm were cut, making it impossible for me to use it, and the lung deflated and tubes were inserted. This type of major surgery, of course, altered the left breast dramatically. The diagnosis was fibrosarcoma of the chest wall. This left me with intolerable chest pain for the rest of my life, which would be complicated by injuries and scar tissue growth. Following the 11 hours of surgery, I was told that I would have a maximum of two months to live and that they would keep me as comfortable as possible. "You have cancer! Not only cancer, but one of the deadliest forms of bone cancer, with no possibility of survival." Remember, this was is in 1970. Today, advances have been made, but the outcome still depends on each individual case. There you have it. The dreaded death sentence that everyone associates with the disease of cancer. Today, things have changed and instead of an automatic death sentence, we now ask, "What is my survival chance?"

I hope telling my story will give it a purpose far beyond my own existence. Maybe my suffering and all the survival techniques I learned as a result can help lessen some of the emotional burdens of others. My aim is to help everyone touched by this dreaded disease. You do not need to have the disease personally to become its victim. It can affect anyone who is in your world. I have attempted to take the loss and destruction that cancer caused me and turn it around. All of what I have been through made me strong beyond my years and tolerant of the many acts in life that usually elicit anger. My outlook is that all things can be wonderful—this smile, this touch, even pain and disappointment can give me a high because my alternative was not to be here at all. Make cancer give you more than it can take away.

When I received the news that I had cancer, I thought my world had just come to an end. *My God, what am I supposed to do? I have three small babies at home and a whole life ahead of me. I don't have time for this, nor do I want to be so frightened. Please don't tell me that I am going to die. Please don't tell me that I am going to suffer beyond anything that I could imagine. Please don't take my world away from me and replace it with a living hell until such time that I exist no longer on this earth.* Always we ask the question, "Why has this happened to me? What did I ever do to deserve this?" For these questions, there are no answers. We are not punished by having this dreaded disease, we only have it by chance.

Because of cancer, I learned to enjoy, respect, achieve, console, know great fulfillment and gain extreme insight into what is really important in this life. Too many people make the mistake of judging life by its length rather than by its depth, or by its problems rather than its promises. We have no say over the hand dealt us in life, but we do have a lot of control over how this hand is played. We are all responsible for bringing out the meaning of our own lives in each moment that we live. Remember each moment happens only once and can never be retrieved again. Everything we are, or are remembered for, revolves around our choices and our actions. Many times I have said, "I have been truly blessed throughout my life *because* I had the dreaded disease of cancer."

Roberta Andresen

Fifty Things I've Learned Along the Way

- I've learned that nursing is the hardest and easiest thing I've ever done.
- I've learned to take my job seriously but myself lightly.
- I've learned that every day I've held a hand but forgotten to chart vital signs I still may have come out ahead.
- I've learned that nursing is extraordinary because we do ordinary things so magnificently.
- I've learned that if I don't get emotionally involved with my patients, it's time for me to change professions.
- I've learned that when you're 92, you shouldn't have to beg for the salt shaker even if you have congestive heart failure.
- I've learned that a patient doesn't get cancer, a family does.
- I've learned that a good physician is one who will say, "I have no idea what's going on with this patient, come help me figure it out."

- I've learned to help people see the "gift of cancer."
- I've learned that if my child tells me she has a bake sale tomorrow at 8 A.M., to be thankful that it's a bake sale and not a teenage pregnancy meeting.
- I've learned that whatever you need in a hurry will be in someone else's room.
- I've learned that when the narcotic count is off, it's usually I who forgot to sign something out.
- I've learned that healing the spirit is as important as healing the body.
- I've learned that if I don't take care of myself, I can't take care of anyone else.
- I've learned that hospital food must be a punishment for our sins in a previous life.
- I've learned that a body believes every word you tell it.
- I've learned that the nurse I'd like to have take care of the person I love most should be me or you.
- I've learned that time flies whether I'm having fun or not.
- I've learned that reality is what is, not what I would like it to be.
- I've learned that if I can't cure, I can still care.
- I've learned that patient-centered care doesn't mean amenities, it means empowerment.
- I've learned that one of the gentlest things I can do is attend all my patients' funerals.
- I've learned that if I'm there before it's over that I'm still on time.
- I've learned to separate between a minor event and a major episode.
- I've learned that it's usually better to beg forgiveness than to ask permission, especially if I'm taking a St. Bernard to see a child in ICU.
- I've learned that good nurses aren't measured as much by punctuality as by compassion.

- I've learned that the spirit of the law may be more important than the letter of the law.
- I've learned that every day I can make a difference in someone's life, and that I choose to make it a positive difference.
- I've learned that if I don't celebrate the exquisiteness of each day, I've lost something I'll never get back.
- I've learned that what helps most when diagnosing patients is never walk behind or ahead of them, but rather walk with them and listen very carefully.
- I've learned that the more unloving a patient acts, the more he or she needs to be loved.
- I've learned that knowing when to stop treatment with a morbidly ill patient may be more important than knowing when to continue.
- I've learned that some things have to be believed to be seen.
- I've learned that addiction to pain medication is the least of our problems when a patient is in pain.
- I've learned that professionals give advice, but healers share wisdom.
- I've learned that meditation, group work, nutritional savvy and massage are as integral to a cancer patient's care as radiation, surgery and chemotherapy.
- I've learned that wearing red polka-dot underwear under my uniform may not be the best choice.
- I've learned that grief knows no rules.
- I've learned that there is no room for bullies or whiners in nursing.
- I've learned that you don't have to meet all the objectives to learn a whole bunch.
- I've learned that a nurse without a sense of humor should try to find a job as a shepherd.

- I've learned that having to work two weekends in a row is a minor event when my breast biopsy comes back benign.
- I've learned that I can work with almost any body fluid but mucus.
- I've learned that student nurses will do something every day that I didn't think was possible.
- I've learned that no one promises us tomorrow.
- I've learned that medical students get anxious when I assign them nursing care or try to see if their chakras are open.
- I've learned that if a confused patient accuses me of "poo-pooing" in his bed, I should apologize and promise never to do it again.
- I've learned that no one says on his death bed, "I wish I'd spent more time at the office."
- I've learned that if a child is old enough to love, she is old enough to grieve.
- I've learned that a lot of patients get well in spite of us, but even more get well because of us.

Sally P. Karioth, Ph.D., R.N.

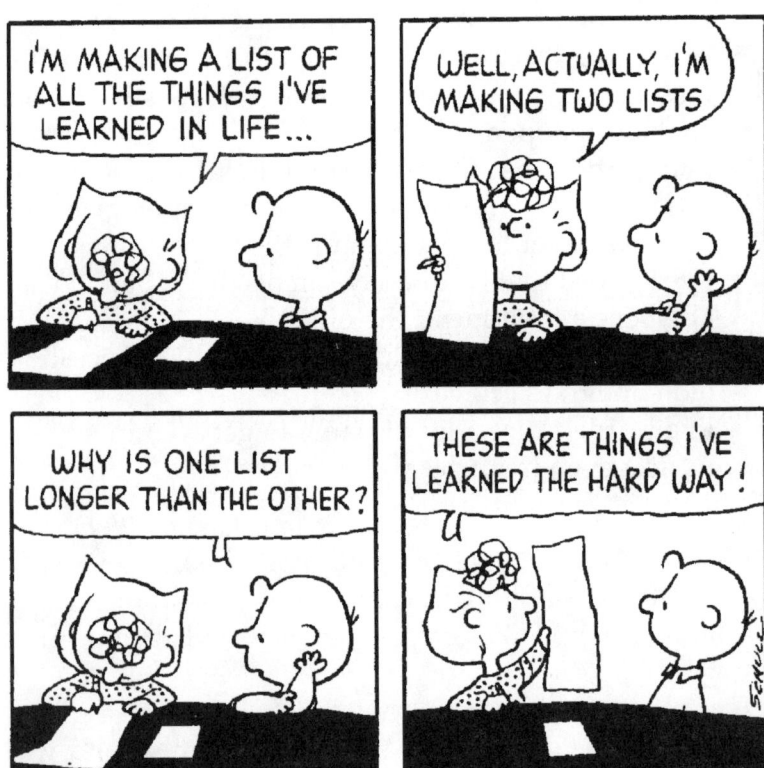

How to Beat Cancer

Today, cancer is the most treatable of all chronic diseases. Half of those diagnosed this year will live out their normal life span, while over 2 million living Americans are now considered cured of cancer. If you have cancer, here are some specific ideas for making your treatment a success.

1. Confront Your Fears.

Cancer evokes powerful negative emotions: Fear that you are losing control over your body and your life. Anger that this is happening. Depression over what you must endure.

For people with cancer, these are all normal feelings. Suppressing them serves only to magnify them and will not help you get better. The way to confront your fears is with education, understanding, faith, positive visualization and relaxation techniques.

Early on, connect with others who have been through the same experience (ask your doctor or hospital about patient support groups).

2. Take Charge.

The leader of your treatment team is you. And the first rule with serious cancer is, get a second opinion. Your current doctor is usually happy to recommend someone, or you can research physicians whom you feel are experts in your cancer.

Take a close friend or relative along to consultations with you. Think in advance of questions you may want to ask, and have your companion take notes for review later (just advise the doctor beforehand). It's hard to deal with your emotions and absorb complex information at the same time.

3. Know Your Options.

Learn as much as you can about your particular kind of cancer—become an expert. It sounds obvious, but try to find out what the latest and most effective treatments are *before* you commit to treatment. (Most physicians are reluctant to change a course of therapy once you've started.)

Centers designated by the National Cancer Institute share the latest information with each other nationwide and can generally offer the newest options and the most advanced treatments.

4. Fight Back.

Keep asking questions throughout treatment and don't take anything for granted. Make sure that you have a doctor, a hospital and a treatment plan *you* feel confident in—don't just take someone else's recommendations on trust.

Don't worry about being a pest: experience shows that patients who aren't intimidated by their disease are the ones most likely to get better.

Don't think solely in terms of medical treatment. You may also need help with family, financial and spiritual issues.

Above all, don't lose your sense of humor. Every day, look for a little pleasure and enjoyment to offset the hours consumed by treatment.

*City of Hope**

---

* The City of Hope has been treating people with cancer for 50 years and is a Clinical Cancer Research Center designated by the National Cancer Institute. We know cancer and will take the time to help you. If you or someone you know has been recently diagnosed, call 1-800-826-HOPE to find out more about treatment available at the City of Hope. For general information about cancer, contact their CancerConnections® hotline at 1-800-678-9990. Cancer doesn't care. We do.®(If you would like to reproduce "How to Beat Cancer" for any purpose, please call the City of Hope at 818-359-8111.)

Celebrate Life!

What lies behind us and what lies before us us are small matter compared to what lies within us.

Ralph Waldo Emerson

Dear Mercy Hospital Patients, Employees and Visitors:

In early June, I was the speaker at our annual National Cancer Survivor Day picnic. This year's theme was *CELEBRATE LIFE.* I took each letter and found a concept to suit it. When I shared the outline of my talk with Mary, my niece, she replied, "Aunt Sue, what you said can apply to anyone—not just people with cancer." Thus, I share CELEBRATE LIFE.

COUNT YOUR BLESSINGS, NOT YOUR WORRIES.
I found this on a little prayer card. It doesn't mean that worries won't come, but when they do, just don't count them. Focus on blessings instead. Choose to see a glass half full, not half empty.

Express your feelings honestly.
Cancer evokes varied emotional reactions. Respect whatever they are honestly. Above all, stay real, concentrating on what's best for you. Don't try to please others by hiding authentic feelings in order to make others feel better.

Learn to laugh and laugh to learn.
Someone once said that laughter is the best medicine. It is! I've come to believe that a sense of humor is as vital as the first five senses (sight, touch, taste, smell, hearing). Having a positive attitude doesn't require smiling all the time, but there is a definite link between our basic attitude and our immune system that is too important to ignore.

Endure what is necessary.
Yes, there's tough stuff in your coping with disease. But never forget the patient who told me her mother always said, "From the day that you're born 'til they take you in a hearse, things are never so bad that they couldn't be worse."

Be open and flexible . . . go with the flow.
Find meaning in the day-by-day doings because little things mean a lot. Ponder the adage, "They who have a why to live can bear almost any how." Cancer is a wake-up call that jolts us out of our complacency.

Remain in charge by networking with family and doctors.
Work with doctors not as a victim but as a partner. Trust your body signals for better or worse. You have a

right to retain an appropriate degree of control in what's happening.

ACCEPT AND FACE YOUR MORTALITY.

This can be a slow and painful process that takes time and effort. Cancer does provide a new awareness of life's previous quality through its unique lens. Death is certain for all of us, but how we live out our remaining days is up to us.

TREASURE EACH DAY AND EACH NEW EXPERIENCE.

No, I wouldn't have chosen cancer on the menu of health struggles, but I would not trade all I've learned, lived, laughed and loved because of it. One marvelous side effect has been connection with incredibly beautiful people. I believe you can turn your back on negativity that wants to drag you down.

EXERCISE BODY, MIND AND SPIRIT AS ABLE.

In the new book, Remarkable Recovery, *by Caryle Hirshberg and Marc Ian Barasch, seven common factors among the survivors are discussed: the will to live, acceptance of the disease but not the outcome, working with doctors as collaborators, having supportive people around, improving diet, exercising more, and finding faith important in recovery.*

LIVE REMEMBERING THAT LIFE IS A MYSTERY TO BE LIVED, NOT A PROBLEM TO BE SOLVED.

As you search for answers, reasons, whys and why nots, remember there is a dimension of all this that remains a mystery. Sometimes health struggles invite us to reverence instead of grueling analysis.

INVEST IN YOUR INNER RESOURCES: COURAGE, EFFORT, DETERMINATION, FAITH, HOPE AND LOVE.
All of these nurture the will to live and flourish. Surprise yourself by opting to maximize who you are by practicing these virtuous behaviors.

FIND THE FUTURE IN YOUR NOW.
Maybe you've wondered if you'd make it today—you're here! Select short-term goals as your ongoing link to life. Meditate on the "Family Circus" cartoon that says, "Yesterday's the past, tomorrow's the future, but today is a gift. That's why it's called the present." Sink your heart into that one.

EMERGE AS A WINNER—NOT A VICTIM OR MERE SURVIVOR, BUT TRULY A THRIVER!
Need I say more? Onward and upward!

Sister Sue Tracy, O.P.

Intravenous Chicken Soup for the Soul™

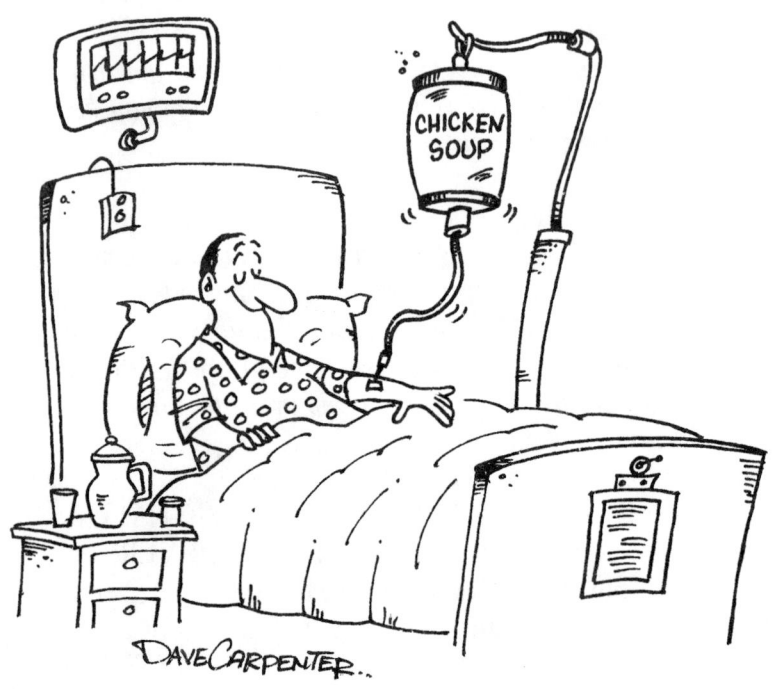

Reprinted with permission from Dave Carpenter.

If you too would like to *intravenously* provide *Chicken Soup* to cancer patients, you can!

For every $12.95 you donate, we will send *Chicken Soup for the Surviving Soul* to one of the listed organizations in our resource section. In addition, we will award 10 percent of the proceeds to The Wellness Community, founded by Dr. Harold Benjamin who continues to be an asset and an inspiration to the cancer community.

Make checks payable to:
Self-Esteem Seminars
P.O. Box 30880
Santa Barbara, CA 93130

More Chicken Soup?

Many of the stories and poems that you have read in this book were submitted by readers such as yourself who responded to our request for stories or sent them in after reading the first three volumes of *Chicken Soup for the Soul.* So we invite you, too, to share a story, poem or article that you feel belongs in a future volume of *Chicken Soup for the Surviving Soul.* This may be a story you clip out of the local newspaper, a magazine, a church bulletin or a hospital newsletter. It might be something you read in a book or receive over the fax, or that favorite quotation you have on the refrigerator door. It could be a poem you have written or your own personal experience that you believe will touch others.

In addition to future editions of *Chicken Soup for the Surviving Soul,* we are going to publish other *Chicken Soup for the Soul* books every year. We are planning special collections of *Chicken Soup* for teachers, parents, women, salespeople, Christians, Jews, teenagers, athletes, animal lovers and people at work. We also plan to have a special volume of humorous stories entitled *Chicken Soup for the Laughing Soul* as well as a collection of Christmas stories.

Just send a copy of your stories and other pieces to us at this address.

Chicken Soup for the Soul
P.O. Box 30880
Santa Barbara, CA 93130
fax: 805-563-2945
e-mail: soup4soul@aol.com

We will be sure that both you and the author are credited for your submission. (In order that we may properly credit the material, please be sure to include the source from which your submission was acquired.) Thank you for your contribution.

Who Is Jack Canfield?

Jack Canfield is one of America's leading experts in the development of human potential and personal effectiveness. He is both a dynamic and entertaining speaker and a highly sought-after trainer, with a wonderful ability to inform and inspire audiences toward increased levels of self-esteem and peak performance.

He is the author and narrator of several bestselling audio- and videocassette programs, including *Chicken Soup for the Soul—Live, Self-Esteem and Peak Performance, How to Build High Self-Esteem* and *Self-Esteem in the Classroom.* He is regularly seen on television shows such as *Good Morning America, 20/20, Eye to Eye* and *NBC Nightly News.* He has coauthored 10 books, including *Chicken Soup for the Soul, A 2nd Helping of Chicken Soup for the Soul, A 3rd Serving of Chicken Soup for the Soul, Chicken Soup for the Soul Cookbook, Dare to Win* and *The Aladdin Factor* (all with Mark Victor Hansen), *100 Ways to Build Self-Concept in the Classroom* (with Harold C. Wells) and *Heart at Work* (with Jacqueline Miller).

Jack speaks regularly to professional associations, school districts, government agencies, churches, hospitals, sales organizations and corporations. His clients have included the American Dental Association, the American Management Association, AT&T, Campbell Soup, Clairol, Domino's Pizza, G.E., ITT Hartford Insurance, Johnson & Johnson, the Million Dollar Roundtable, NCR, New England Telephone, Re/Max, Scott Paper, TRW and Virgin Records. Jack is also on the faculties of two schools for entrepreneurs—Income Builders International and the Life Success Academy.

Jack conducts an annual eight-day Training of Trainers program in the areas of self-esteem and peak performance. It attracts educators, counselors, parenting trainers, corporate trainers, professional speakers, ministers and others interested in developing their speaking and seminar-leading skills.

For further information about Jack's books, tapes and trainings, or to schedule him for a presentation, please write to:

The Canfield Training Group
P.O. Box 30880
Santa Barbara , CA 93130
Call toll free 800-237-8336 or fax 805-563-2945

Who Is Mark Victor Hansen?

Mark Victor Hansen is a professional speaker who in the last 20 years has talked to over one million people in 32 countries, making over 4,000 presentations in the areas of sales excellence and strategies, and personal empowerment and development.

Mark has spent a lifetime dedicated to his mission to make a profound and positive difference in people's lives. Throughout his career, he has inspired hundreds of thousands of people to create more powerful and purposeful futures for themselves while stimulating the sale of billions of dollars worth of goods and services.

Mark has written numerous books, including *Future Diary, How to Achieve Total Prosperity* and *The Miracle of Tithing,* and he has coauthored several books, including *Chicken Soup for the Soul, A 2nd Helping of Chicken Soup for the Soul, A 3rd Serving of Chicken Soup for the Soul, Chicken Soup for the Soul Cookbook, Dare to Win* and *The Aladdin Factor* (all with Jack Canfield).

As well as speaking and writing, Mark has produced a complete library of personal empowerment cassette and video programs that enable his listeners to recognize and use their innate abilities in their business and personal lives. His message has also made him a popular television and radio personality, with appearances on ABC, NBC, CBS and HBO.

Mark has also appeared on the cover of numerous magazines, including *Success* and *Changes. Success* reported his achievements on the cover of its August 1991 issue.

Mark is a big man with a big heart and a big spirit, an inspiration to all who seek to better themselves.

You can contact Mark by writing:

711 W. 17th Street, #D2
Costa Mesa, CA 92627
or by calling 714-759-9304, or from
outside California, 800-433-2314

Who Is Patty Aubery?

Now vice-president of The Canfield Training Group and Self-Esteem Seminars, Inc., Patty Aubery remembers the early days of Jack Canfield's work—before *Chicken Soup for the Soul* took the country by storm. Jack was still telling these heart-warming stories then, in his trainings, workshops and keynote presentations, which Patty scheduled and coordinated.

Later, she directed the labor of love that went into compiling and editing the original 101 *Chicken Soup* stories, and went on to support the daunting marketing effort and steadfast optimism required to bring it to millions of readers worldwide.

Though Patty can't claim the title of bestselling author, noted authority, or even nationally recognized speaker, over 5 million copies have now been sold of the bestselling books that were brought to print with her unique combination of hard work, judgment and insight.

Recently, Patty coauthored the series' fifth and latest offering, *Chicken Soup for the Surviving Soul*. Of the effort, Patty says, "I'm always encouraged, amazed and humbled by the story-tellers I meet when I work on any *Chicken Soup* book, but the overwhelming courage, enduring faith and profound wisdom I encountered from *Surviving Soul* contributors will stay with me forever."

Patty is married to successful entrepreneur Jeff Aubery and together they have a young son, J.T. Aubery. A native of Southern California and an outstanding asset to Jack Canfield's training organization and the *Chicken Soup* phenomenon, Patty and her family make their home in Santa Barbara. She can be reached at:

The Canfield Training Group
P.O. Box 30880
Santa Barbara, CA 93130
805-563-2935
fax: 805-563-2945

Who Is Nancy Mitchell?

Nancy Mitchell is director of publishing for The Canfield Group. She graduated from Arizona State University in May of 1994 with a Bachelor of Science in Nursing.

After graduation, Nancy worked at Good Samaritan Regional Medical Center in Phoenix, Arizona, in the Cardiovascular Intensive Care Unit. Four months after graduation, Nancy moved back to her native town of Los Angeles. Her sister and coauthor, Patty Aubery, offered her a part-time job working for Jack Canfield and Mark Victor Hansen. Nancy's intentions were to help finish *A 2nd Helping of Chicken Soup for the Soul* and then return to nursing. However, in December of that year, she was asked to continue on full-time at The Canfield Group. Nancy put nursing on hold and became the director of publishing, working closely with Jack and Mark on all *Chicken Soup for the Soul* projects.

Nancy says that right now what she is most thankful for is her move back to L.A. "If I hadn't moved back to California, I wouldn't have had the chance to be there for my mom during her bout with breast cancer. Right now my priority is to be there for my mom and for my family."

Nancy has recently relocated to Santa Barbara with The Canfield Group and can be reached at:

The Canfield Group
P.O. Box 30880
Santa Barbara, CA 93130
800-237-8336
fax: 805-563-2945

Contributors

Many of the stories in this book were taken from books we have read. These sources are acknowledged in the Permissions section. Most of the stories and poems were contributed by cancer survivors, many of whom are professional speakers. If you would like to contact them for information on their books, tapes and seminars, you can reach them at the address and phone numbers provided below.

Many of the stories were also contributed by readers like yourself, who responded to our request for stories. We have included information about them as well.

Roberta Andresen has been active in the business world her whole adult life, holding positions ranging from clerical to managerial. She is the author of *My Daddy Died*. She is available to speak to any size group and can be reached by calling 800-749-2550.

Maggie Bedrosian is a business owner and executive coach, specializing in helping people produce focused results with natural ease. She is the author of three books, including *Life Is More Than Your To-Do List: Blending Business Success with Personal Satisfaction*. Maggie is the past president of the American Society for Training and Development, Washington, D.C., chapter, and also chaired the Writing/Publishing Group of the National Speakers Association. You can contact Maggie by calling 301-460-3408.

Harold H. Benjamin, Ph.D., conceived of the breakthrough "patient active" concept based on his experience in dealing with psychological and emotional aspects of cancer. He founded The Wellness Community in 1982 as a no-cost program for cancer patients. Harold can be reached at The Wellness Community—National, 2716 Ocean Park Blvd., Suite 1040, Santa Monica, CA 90405, 310-314-2555

Louise Biggs is married and has three sons. When her older sons were in college, she decided to join them and received her teaching degree in 1982 at the age of 42. She has been teaching fifth grade for 13 years. She enjoys an active church life, camping, hiking, quilting, basket weaving, and doll-making. She can be reached at 4616 Old Stage Rd., Pulaski, VA 24301, or call 540-980-4016.

Linda Blackman is president of Executive Image, Inc. She is a former national television anchor, reporter and talk show host. Today she is a sought-after professional speaker and trainer to businesses and associations. Linda uses her unique methods to show you how to enhance your image by winning every audience. Contact her at 5020 Castleman St., Pittsburgh, PA 15232, or call 412-682-2200.

William M. Buchholz, M.D., is an oncologist and a graduate of Harvard and Stanford. William is in practice with his wife, Susan, a clinical psychologist, in Mountain View, California. He is a consultant to the Commonweal Cancer Help Program in Bolinas, California. In his oncology practice he combines conventional and complementary therapies, with an emphasis on empowering patients and their families. He has found that a little hope goes a long way.

Diana L. Chapman has been a newspaper journalist for more than 11 years, having worked at *The Los Angeles Times, The San Diego Union* and Los Angeles Copley Newspapers. She specializes in touching human interest stories and, after being diagnosed with multiple sclerosis in 1993, began working on a book involving health issues. She has been married for seven years and has one son, Herbert Ryan Hart. She can be reached by calling 310-548-1192 or writing to 837 Elberon #3A, San Pedro, CA 90731.

Dianne Clark is a business education teacher at Castleford High School in Castleford, Idaho. She lives on the family farm with her husband, Ted, and teenage sons, Russ and Nic. Dianne enjoys making various craft items and is committed to Twelve-Step Recovery. You can contact Dianne at 1000 E. 3211 N., Buhl, ID 83316, or call 208-537-6821.

Reverend Robert Craig is a United Methodist minister. From 1980 to 1994, he was a chaplain at Methodist Medical Center in Peoria, Illinois, where he served as a surgical chaplain and worked with the open-heart team. Reverend Craig can be reached at 102 South Niles, Metamora, IL 61548.

Janine Crawford is a bookkeeper for a real estate firm in Arcadia, California. Her first love is children; she loves creating children's clothing and baby quilts. After graduating from high school, she attended the Institute for Design and Merchandising in Los Angeles. Her artwork is now an enjoyable hobby. This is her first attempt at writing.

Christine M. Creley is a first-grade teacher and lives with her husband, Terry, in Memphis, Tennessee. Her interests include travel, reading and aerobics. She can be reached by writing 3904 Robin Hill Dr., Bartlett, TN 38135.

Sally deLipkau is the oncology patient representative for Washoe Medical Center and assists cancer patients and families both individually and in group settings. She provides communitywide presentations for the early detection of breast cancer as well as inspirational presentations. Sally trains volunteers and coordinates programs for the American Cancer Society and is a hospice volunteer.

Manuel Diotte contracted cancer at the age of seven and was given six months to live. After 26 operations, two years of chemotherapy and several months of radiation treatment, Manuel overcame these seemingly insurmountable odds. He is 27 years old today and considers himself a walking miracle. Through radio and TV, Manuel has inspired countless individuals with his stories about love, hope, faith and courage. Manuel is now a professional speaker and businessman who resides in San Antonio with his wife, Heather. You can contact Manuel at 314 Cypressfox, San Antonio, TX 78245, or call 210-681-7527.

Joanne P. Freeman is an attorney and a writer. She holds a B.A. in literature from the University of Arizona and a law degree from the University of California, Davis. She has previously published essays, film critiques and book reviews in *The Los Angeles Daily News, The Los Angeles Daily Journal* and *The Wall Street Journal's National Business Employment Weekly*. Joanne can be reached at 2220 Miraval Tercero, Tucson, AZ 85718, or call 520-299-6172.

Howard J. Fuerst, M.D., received his medical degree from the University of Pennsylvania in 1949. He spent two years in the U.S. Air Force and then entered the practice of internal medicine in Hollywood, Florida. He retired from this practice in 1986. In 1991, he became interested in alternative medicine and today conducts a cancer support group. He has and will continue to espouse alternative medicine modalities to any forum.

Katherine Stephens Gallagher was employed in the human resources department of Harris Methodist Hospital when she was diagnosed with breast cancer in April 1992. She underwent a double mastectomy with reconstruction. She dedicates a majority of her time to working with the American Cancer Society, serving on the Doris Kupferele Advisory Board at Harris Methodist Hospital and also as a Reach to Recovery volunteer. Katherine finds working with other women who face this disease to be most rewarding and gratifying. She can be reached at 7120 Serrano Dr., Fort Worth, TX 76126, or call 817-731-0526.

Katie Gill is a senior English major at John Carroll University in Cleveland, Ohio, and will be graduating in May 1996. She plans to pursue a career in writing and eventually wants to write a book about what it was like having cancer at the age of 16, in order to offer hope to other teenagers with cancer. Katie can be reached at 4520 Ashbury Park Dr., North Olmstead, OH 44070, or call 216-777-7726.

Katie Griffler is 14 years old and loves art, writing, drawing and acting. She especially loves dance and helping others. She has three brothers, two dogs and a three-legged cat. Katie says her mother is her inspiration for everything and her dad is a great guy who spoils her rotten. She can be reached at 6 Carbury Rd., Ocean, NJ 07712, or call 908-493-3171.

Jane Hill is a breast cancer survivor and a member of the 1995-96 National Cancer Survivors' Speakers Bureau. A comedienne, she delivers keynote speeches and presents workshops on humor and health. She has performed nationwide for thousands of cancer survivors and healthcare professionals, and has been featured on various television programs on humor and healing.

Jane also serves on the board of the Orange County chapter of the Susan G. Komen Breast Cancer Foundation. Additionally, she and her 15-year-old daughter, Kelly, helped to start the Komen Kids' program in 1993—a friendship and support network for kids who have a parent with cancer, and now a national program sponsored by the Komen Foundation. Jane can be reached by writing 3941 South "E" Bristol St., Suite 337, Santa Ana, CA 92704 or by calling 714-546-2339.

Sally P. Karioth, Ph.D., R.N., is a professor at Florida State University, where she teaches "Death, the Individual Family." For more than 20 years she has been a counselor, helping people cope with the death of loved ones, particularly parents who have lost a child to death. You can contact Sally by writing Living Is Fun Enterprises, 2406 Mexia Ave., Tallahassee, FL 32304 or by calling 904-575-9394.

Wanda Kelly, together with her late husband, Orville Kelly, founded two national organizations: Make Today Count, a grass-roots, self-help organization for persons with life-threatening illnesses; and the National Association of Atomic Veterans, to help those sickened by exposure to atomic testing. After her husband's death in 1980, she continued their shared mission of helping others by traveling on behalf of both organizations. Wanda lives in Osage Beach, Missouri. She received her Realtor's license and sells property in the beautiful Lake of the Ozarks for Four Seasons Shores Realty.

Maureen Khan-Lacoss is the mother of the two most wonderful blessings in her life, Matthew and Johnathan, to whom she would like to dedicate her story for their May birthdays. Maureen says the reason for her being positive in the face of losing her leg to cancer 25 years ago is due to her mom and dad, Maureen and Duran, who are the reason she is who she is! Maureen can be reached by writing P.O. Box 212, Quaker Hill, CT 06375.

Chris King is a human-development specialist, artist, storyteller, trainer, consultant, TV announcer, aerobics instructor, model, mathematician, salesperson, waitress, newspaper editor, writer, speaker and mother of five. Chris' mission is to help others exercise their innate creativity in order to improve the quality of their personal and work lives. "Creativity is not only a necessity today, it is fun, energizing and rewarding!" she tells us. Chris can be reached at P.O. Box 221255, Beachwood, OH 44122, or call 216-991-8428.

Kristine Kirsten grew up in Los Angeles and was raised by her mother. She likes to read, write, play acoustic and electric guitars, and work out at the gym. Besides pursuing an acting career and writing a book about her battle with cancer, she would like to attend nursing school so that she can comfort patients the way nurses have comforted her.

Allen Klein (a.k.a. Mr. Jollytologist) is a professional speaker and bestselling author. As a recipient of a Toastmasters award and a Certified Speaking Professional designation from the National Speakers Association, he shows audiences nationwide how to find humor in not-so-funny stuff. Allen is also the author of *The Healing Power of Humor, Quotations to Cheer You Up When the World Is Getting You Down* and *Wing Tips*. His mother is very proud of him. Allen can be reached by writing 1034 Page St., San Francisco, CA 94117 or by calling 415-431-1913.

Paula (Bachleda) Koskey is a happy soul surviving well in Berkley, Michigan. Her main pleasures consist of her three children (currently at the "hormone hostages" stage, a.k.a. teenagers), jogging, reading and chocolate. She's a firm believer in SRAK (Sneaky Random Acts of Kindness) and delights in thinking of devious and mischievous ways of spreading smiles. She also enjoys speaking and writing and has written a children's book, *Secrets of Christmas*. Paula can be reached by writing 1173 Cambridge, Berkley, MI 48072.

Peter Legge is the president and CEO of Canada Wide Magazines and Communications. This organization publishes 19 magazines across Canada and worth over $20 million in sales. Peter travels worldwide speaking to over 100 organizations annually. He has authored the books, *How to Soar with the Eagles* and *You Can If You Believe You Can*. Toastmasters International has honored Peter with two awards, the Golden Gavel and the Top Speaker in North America. You can reach him by writing Peter Legge Management Co. Ltd., 4th Floor, 4180 Lougheed Hwy, Burnaby, BC V5C 6A7.

Gregory M. Lousig-Nont, Ph.D., is the president of Lousig-Nont & Associates, an 18-year-old human resource potential consulting firm. He conducts motivational seminars and his new book, *Habits of Happiness: The Book That Answers the Question, If I'm So Damn Happy Why Does My Life Suck?*, is scheduled for release in the summer of 1996. Gregory can be reached at 3740 Royal Crest St., Las Vegas, NV 89119, or call 1-800-477-3211.

Cynthia Bonney Mannering, M.A.T., educates others about support for cancer patients. The compassion and care she received from professionals, friends and family during her bone marrow transplant were key to her survival. Her own story, extensive public speaking experience, and research on caregiving make her a warm and inspiring speaker/consultant. To contact her for speaking engagements, or to contribute your own suggestions for the love and care of cancer patients, write to 810 Warm Springs Ave., Boise, ID 83712 or call 208-385-9855.

Hanoch McCarty, Ed.D., is a dynamic, entertaining and internationally known speaker, educational psychologist, and author. His motivational keynote addresses, seminars and workshops for major corporations, conventions, professional associations, schools and parent groups are noted for their high energy, great humor, participant involvement and perceptive insights. He is the author of 14 books and audio training programs, including *Acts of Kindness: How to Create a Kindness Revolution* and *A Year of Kindness: 365 Ways to Spread Sunshine*. He has been a frequent guest on radio and television programs all over the U.S. He can be reached by writing P.O. Box 66, Galt, CA 95632 or by calling 209-745-2212.

Meladee Dawn McCarty is a dynamic speaker on topics r૨
esteem, deliberate kindness programs and innovative approa૮..
education. She is a program specialist at the Sacramento County Office ૦૧
Education. She finds placements for severely handicapped children and
works extensively with their families and teachers. She is the coauthor, with
Hanoch McCarty, of *Acts of Kindness: How to Create a Kindness Revolution*. She can
be reached by writing P.O. Box 66, Galt, CA 95632 or by calling 209-745-2212.

Susan Chernak McElroy has been an animal lover all of her life. She has
worked with animals for years as a veterinarian's assistant, humane society
educator, dog trainer, wildlife rehabilitator and zookeeper. McElroy's vision
is to heal the relationship between people and animals. She makes her home
in Oregon at Bright Star Farm. She can be reached at NewSage Press, P.O. Box
607, Troutdale, OR 97060-0607 or fax 503-695-5406.

Lisa McKeehan is a kindergarten teacher in La Jolla, California. She graduated
from Loyola Marymount University in 1993. In 1994, she received her teaching
credential and cross-cultural language and academic certificate, enabling her to
teach students from a variety of diverse ethnic and language backgrounds. Lisa
also received her master's degree in curriculum and instruction, with a literacy
emphasis, in December 1995. She began volunteering for Camp Ronald
McDonald in 1994 and plans to continue at every opportunity.

Peter McWilliams is the author and coauthor of several books, including *How
to Survive the Loss of a Love; You Can't Afford the Luxury of a Negative Thought; How
to Heal Depression; Do It! Let's Get Off Our Butts; Life 101; Life 102: What to Do When
Your Guru Sues You;* and *Ain't Nobody's Business If You Do: The Absurdity of
Consensual Crime in a Free Country*. Most of his books are available for free
browsing on the internet at http://www.mcwilliams.com.

Mary Lyn Miller, a communications consultant, teacher, speaker and writer,
is the founder of The Career Clinic. A former corporate executive, Mary Lyn
had to first heal herself. While recovering from cancer, she designed a breakthrough process for life direction which affected the lives of thousands of
people who have sought to embrace their dreams and be all they are
designed to be. She can be reached at 3901 Highland Ave., Suite 2,
Manhattan Beach, CA 90266, 310-545-8717.

Jann Mitchell is the author of three books: *Home Sweeter Home: Creating a
Haven of Simplicity and Spirit, Codependent for Sure! An Original Jokebook* and
Organized Serenity. Her popular column, "Relating," about our relationships
with ourselves and others, runs Sundays in *The Oregonian* in Portland and in
newspapers around the country. The award-winning journalist is a sought-
after speaker on self-development and simplifying one's life. Jann can be
reached by writing 7714-C SW Barnes Rd., Portland, OR 97225 or by calling
503-221-8516.

Linda Mitchell is the mother of two of this book's coauthors, Patty Mitchell
Aubery and Nancy Mitchell. Linda was diagnosed with breast cancer in

January 1995. She underwent seven weeks of radiation and a lumpectomy and today is cancer-free. Linda works full-time with her son-in-law, manufacturing golf bags. During her free time, Linda enjoys golfing, walking, reading and spending a few weeks out of the year with her husband, Terry, in Maui. Cancer taught Linda that you only live once and life should be enjoyed to the fullest. She can be reached by calling 818-368-2364.

Marilyn Moody is currently employed by the Orange County Department of Social Services. She is single and the grandmother of three. Writing has become a major part of her life since the cancer diagnosis. Her leisure time is now being used to finish a play, *Love and Laughter,* about her on-line cancer group. Upon completion, it will be performed by the Teaneck New Theater in New Jersey. Marilyn can be reached by calling 714-848-0800.

P. S. Mueller is a cartoon artist whose work has appeared in *The Chicago Reader, The Austin Chronicle, Utne Reader, Harper's Magazine* and scores of other publications over the past 25 years. His cartoons are featured daily in the *Green Bay Press-Gazette* and are published in numerous college newspapers. Mueller lives and works in Madison, Wisconsin.

Claire Nuer cofounded the ACC International Institute in 1989, a non-profit organization offering educational programs worldwide for those concerned by life-threatening or chronic illnesses, and for anyone who wants to improve the quality and vigor of his or her life. ACC's activities include training programs, conferences, seminars and ongoing support in the fields of health, education, human resources and intercultural dialogue. ACC stands for Au Coeur de la Communication (At the Heart of Communication). Claire can be reached by writing ACC International Institute, P.O. Box 335, Corte Madera, CA 94976 or by calling 415-789-8802.

Erik Olesen is a professional speaker, psychotherapist and author who helps people become more confident, relaxed and productive. He has spoken for over 80 organizations throughout North America. Olesen's book, Mastering the Winds of Change: Peak Performers Reveal How to Stay on Top in Times of Turmoil (HarperCollins) features a complete conditioning program for mastering the pressure of change in the 1990s and beyond. His book for children, *The Little Sailboat and the Big Storm* (Coming of Age Press), helps kids become more confident and optimistic. To order books, or to contact Erik Olesen, please write to 2740 Fulton, Suite 203, Sacramento, CA 95821, or call toll-free 800-STRONG-U.

Eileen Brown O'Riley was born in Brooklyn, New York, and has overcome many obstacles, including breast cancer and surgery. Since the time of her surgery, with the help of a devoted husband and supportive, loving family, she has come through her trauma a much stronger person. She chose the subject of her mastectomy as a thesis topic when she returned to school to complete her master's degree in education.

Bernadette Randle is a former professional pianist and arranger and now serves as music director for the New Life Family Church. Bernadette teaches piano, tutors students in English composition and math, and is a graphic illustrator for the U.S. Army. She is a voracious reader, an inspirational speaker, and a comedic personality who currently aspires to "qualify for AARP membership." Bernadette can be contacted at P.O. Box 1732, Maryland Heights, MO, or call 314-576-5972.

Mary L. Rapp was born in New York. She is the oldest of 12 children which she says prepared her well for motherhood and a career in nursing—both of which she has enjoyed immensely. Mary loves dogs, collects teacups, is an avid reader and keeps a journal. She says cancer has been the greatest challenge of her life.

Rachel Naomi Remen, M.D., is one of the pioneers of Mind/Body/Spirit medicine. She is the assistant clinical professor of family and community medicine at the UCSF School of Medicine and cofounder and medical director of the Commonweal Cancer Retreat featured on Bill Moyers' PBS special *Healing and the Mind*. She has been a cancer therapist for 20 years. Her new book *Kitchen Table Wisdom* will be published by Riverhead in September 1996.

Nancy Rihard-Guilford is a professional speaker specializing in interactive workshops on self-esteem, optimum performance and creating a joyful life. No Johnny-come-lately to the field, her teaching of self-esteem dates back to 1980. Known for her humor and practical strategies, her client list ranges from metaphysical churches to the United States Navy. She is the author of the upcoming *Yikes!—Time for Plan B*. You can contact Nancy at P.O. Box 24220, Ventura, CA 93002 or call 805-648-6590.

Adrienne Rivera graduated from the University of Colorado with a degree in aerospace engineering in December 1992. She was a member of the U.S. Disabled Ski Team from 1990 to 1994. Adrienne competed in the 1994 Olympics in disabled alpine skiing and won a gold and a bronze medal. She was one of 12 Olympians selected to take the Olympic flame to Sarajevo on a peace mission. She made a presentation to President Clinton on behalf of the disabled teams. Adrienne is retired from racing, works as an aerospace engineer in Denver and is pursuing her master's degree in engineering management.

Jaime Rosenthal is a freshman at Pennsylvania State University. Her mother was diagnosed with breast cancer in March 1994 and had a mastectomy and chemotherapy. In November of the same year she underwent a second mastectomy, followed by five weeks of radiation. Today, her hair has grown back completely and she looks and feels wonderful. Jaime can be reached at 848 Weber Dr., Yardley, PA 19067.

David Roth is a singer, songwriter, recording artist, conference presenter, emcee, husband, basketball aficionado, playwright and workshop facilitator. The story "Manuel Garcia" was reported by William Janz in the *Milwaukee*

Sentinel, and the song can be found on David's first recording, *Rising in Love.* He can be reached by writing 18952 40th Place NE, Seattle, WA 98155 or by calling 1-800-484-2367.

Paul Santoro is 54 years old and was raised mostly in the Western United States. He has 3 children. He has become even more thoughtful of the whole human drama since his spiritual experience. It is his feeling that our souls need and want to evolve—and that each of us is on an immense journey to reconcile our will with that of God's. Even with all of the incredible horror of man's inhumanity, Paul still believes in and loves us.

John Wayne Schlatter is a speaker whose topics are inspirational, full of insight and rich with his own special brand of humor. Jack is a former speech and drama teacher as well as an author of many works. His latest book is entitled Gifts By The Side of the Road. Jack was listed in the 1990 edition of Who's Who Among Teachers in America. He is a member of the Professionals Speakers Network. In 1993, he was honored by his peers with the prestigious Speaker of the Year Award. Jack can be reached at P.O. Box 577, Cypress, CA 90630 or by calling 714-879-7271.

Harley L. Schwadron is a former newspaper reporter and public relations writer living and working in Ann Arbor, Michigan. He has been a full-time cartoonist since 1985, specializing in business, health and topical cartoons. His freelance cartoons appear in magazines around the world, and his op-ed work can be seen in such papers as *The Washington Post, The Washington Times, The Dayton Daily News, The Los Angeles Times* and *The Des Moines Register.* For many years he was a regular cartoonist featured in England's *Punch* magazine.

Delva Joan Seavy-Rebin exemplifies the triumph of the human spirit. Robbed of her parents by cancer and afflicted herself, she survived despite a dire prognosis. Willpower has been the strong suit of this indomitable natural scientist, author, professor, mother and wife. Recipient of the U.S. International Ambassador Award (National Speakers Association), the Canadian Citation of Citizenship and her university's Spirit of Youth Award, this 11th-generation North American continues to light the path for others.

Bernie Siegel, M.D., is the author of the bestselling *Love, Medicine and Miracles, Peace, Love and Healing,* and *How to Live Between Office Visits.* Dr. Siegel is deeply involved in humanizing medical education and making the medical profession and patients aware of the mind-body connection. Bernie and his wife, Bobbie, have five children and reside in New Haven, Connecticut. In 1978 Bernie started ECaP, Exceptional Cancer Patients, located at 2 Church Street South, New Haven, CT 06519.

Kimberly A. Stoliker is a two-and-a-half-year survivor of inflammatory breast cancer. She corresponds with women from all over the country who have or have had this type of breast cancer. She is very involved with The Greater Capital District Coalition for Cancer Survivorship in Albany, New York. She is hoping to have a book published that follows her day-to-day treatment in order to help other women who will undergo autologous bone marrow transplants. Kimberly can be reached at 173 Middletown Rd., Waterford, NY 12188 or by calling 518-235-9930.

Sybil Taylor is an author/journalist born in Paris. Some of her works include *The Tellington Touch, The Last Run* and *Ireland's Pubs*. Her most recent article, on Santa Fe, New Mexico, appeared in the May/June 1995 issue of *Endless Vacation*. Sybil remains infinitely grateful for and aware of the precious gifts of life, health and love she continues to enjoy.

Sister Sue Tracy, O.P., is a Grand Rapids Dominican Sister who has been pastoral care director at Mercy Hospital in Toledo, Ohio, since 1989. Prior to this she was a high school teacher, vocation director, religious education director and liturgist. Sister Sue has coped with breast cancer twice and regularly provides public speaking about these experiences. She focuses on being a cancer thriver and not just a survivor. She can be contacted at Mercy Hospital, 2200 Jefferson Ave., Toledo, OH 43624, or call 419-259-1413.

Anne C. Washburn is the cancer patient education coordinator at the North Carolina Clinical Cancer Center in Chapel Hill. She plans, implements and evaluates cancer education and psychosocial programming for oncology patients and their families. In 1988, a year after her mother's death, she decided to volunteer with hospice so she could assist other terminally ill patients. Her personal experience, volunteer time, and academic background in public health led her naturally into oncology. After completing a fellowship at the National Cancer Institute's Office of Cancer Communications, she was fortunate to find a position where she is able to help meet the psychosocial needs of cancer patients and families every day. She can be reached at 919-966-3097.

Bob Westenberg is a leading direct-mail and fundraising copywriter and consultant. He can be reached at 95 Devil's Kitchen Dr., Sedona, AZ 86351, or call 520-284-1111.

Norma Yamamoto resides in Huntington Beach, California, with her husband, Albert, and daughter, Amy. She is happy to report that her son, Brian, is now a sophomore at UCLA and the latest MRI has shown that the tumors are gone and he is in remission! This story was submitted to *Coping* magazine in 1994, and Brian was chosen as the 1995 Coping Cancer Survivor of the Year. Norma can be reached at 17401 Wildrose Ln., Huntington Beach, CA 92649.

Resources

American Brain Tumor Association
2720 River Road, Suite 146
Des Plaines, IL 60018
800-886-2282

American Cancer Society
1599 Clifton Road, NE
Atlanta, GA 30329
800-ACS-2345

**American Institute for
Cancer Research**
1759 R Street NW
Washington, DC 20069
202-328-7744

American Lung Association
1740 Broadway
New York, NY 10019
212-265-5642
212-315-8700 (fax)

**R. A. Bloch Cancer
Foundation, Inc.**
The Cancer Hotline
4410 Main Street
Kansas City, MO 64111
816-932-8543

**Bone Marrow Transplant
Family Support Network**
P.O. Box 845
Avon, CT 06001
800-826-9376

**Bone Marrow Transplant
(BMT) Newsletter**
1985 Spruce Avenue
Highland Park, IL 60035
708-831-1913

Burger King Cancer Caring Center
4117 Liberty Avenue
Pittsburgh, PA 15224
412-622-1212

Cancer Care, Inc.
1180 Avenue of the Americas
New York, NY 10036
212-221-3300

Cancer Conquerors Foundation
P.O. Box 238
Hershey, PA 17033
800-238-6479
717-533-6124

Cancer Research Institute
681 Fifth Avenue
New York, NY 10022
212-688-7515
800-992-2623
212-832-9376 (fax)

Cancer Support Network
Esse House, Suite L10
Baum Blvd. at South Negley
  Avenue
Pittsburgh, PA 15206
412-361-8600

Cancervive
6500 Wilshire Blvd., Suite 500
Los Angeles, CA 90048
310-203-9232

**Candlelighters Childhood
Cancer Foundation**
7910 Woodmont Avenue, Suite 460
Bethesda, MD 20814
800-366-2223
301-657-8401

ChemoCare
231 North Avenue West
Westfield, NJ 07090
800 55-CHEMO (outside NJ)
908-233-1103 (inside NJ)

The Chemotherapy Foundation
183 Madison Avenue, Suite 403
New York, NY 10016
212-213-9292

Children's Oncology Camps
of America
75 Richland Memorial Park
Suite 203
Columbia, SC 29203
803-434-3533

City of Hope Development Center
208 W. 8th Street
Los Angeles, CA 90014
800-835-5504

City of Hope National
Medical Center
1500 E. Duarte Road
Duarte, CA 91010
818-359-8111

Coping Magazine
P.O. Box 682268
Franklin, TN 37068-2268
615-790-2400
615-794-0179 (fax)
E-mail: Copingmag@aol.com

Corporate Angel Network (CAN)
Westchester County Airport
Building 1
White Plains, NY 10604
914-328-1313

ECaP
Exceptional Cancer Patients
2 Church Street South
New Haven, CT 06519

Families Against Cancer (FACT)
P.O. Box 588
DeWitt, NY 13214
315-446-6385
315-446-5326 (fax)

Friends Network
P.O. Box 4545
Santa Barbara, CA 93140
805-565-7031

International Myeloma
Foundation
2120 Stanley Hills Drive
Los Angeles, CA 90046
800-452-CURE

Leukemia Society of America
600 Third Avenue
New York, NY 10016
212-573-8484

Lymphoma Research Foundation
of America, Inc.
2318 Prosser Avenue
Los Angeles, CA 90064
310-470-4912

Make Today Count
Mid-America Cancer Center
1235 E. Cherokee
Springfield, MO 65804
800-432-2273

National Alliance of Breast
Cancer Organizations
9 East 37th Street, 10th Floor
New York, NY 10016
212-719-4154

National Bone Marrow
Transplant Link (BMT Link)
29209 Northwestern Hwy., #624
Southfield, MI 48034
800-LINK-BMT

National Brain Tumor Foundation
785 Market Street, Suite 16
San Francisco, CA 94103
800-934-CURE

National Breast Cancer Coalition
1707 L Street NW, Suite 1060
Washington, DC 21036
202-265-6854
202-296-7477 (fax)

National Cancer Institute Cancer Information Service
Building 31, Room 10A16
9000 Rockville Pike
Bethesda, MD 20892
800-4-CANCER
301-402-5874 (CANCERFAX)

National Cancer Survivors Day Foundation
P.O. Box 682285
Franklin, TN 37068-2285
615-794-3006
615-794-0179 (fax)

National Coalition for Cancer Research
426 C Street NE
Washington, DC 20002
202-544-1880

National Coalition for Cancer Survivorship
1010 Wayne Avenue, 5th Floor
Silver Spring, MD 20910
301-650-8868

National Lymphedema Network
221 I Post Street, Suite 404
San Francisco, CA 94115
800-541-3259

National Marrow Donor Program
3433 Broadway Street NE
Suite 400
Minneapolis, MN 55413
800-MARROW-2

Patient Advocates for Advanced Cancer Treatments
1143 Parmelee NW
Grand Rapids, MI 49504
616-453-1477

Ronald McDonald Houses
One Kroc Drive
Oak Brook, IL 60521
708-575-7418

The Skin Cancer Foundation
245 Fifth Avenue, Suite 2402
New York, NY 10016
212-725-5176

Support for People with Oral and Head and Neck Cancer, Inc.
P.O. Box 53
Locust Valley, NY 11560
516-759-5333

The Wellness Community
2716 Ocean Park Blvd., Suite 1040
Santa Monica, CA 90405
310-314-2555

Y-ME
National Breast Cancer
Organization
212 W. Van Buren, 4th Floor
Chicago, IL 60607
800-221-2141

Permissions *(continued from page iv)*

Wild Bill. Reprinted by permission of Mary L. Rapp. ©1995 Mary L. Rapp.

Kids with Cansur. Reprinted by permission of Random House, Inc. ©1992 Geralyn Gaes, Craig Gaes, and Philip Bashe.

Cancer Has Been a Blessing. Reprinted by permission of Kimberly A. Stoliker. ©1995 Kimberly A. Stoliker.

Cancer and Career Choices. Reprinted by permission of Robert H. Doss. ©1995 Robert H. Doss.

It Is the Best of Times. Reprinted by permission of Joanne P. Freeman. ©1995 Joanne P. Freeman.

Up the Down Slope. Reprinted with permission from *Guideposts Magazine.* ©1988 by Guideposts, Carmel, NY 10512.

Never Give Up! Reprinted by permission of Prentice Hall/Career Development. Excerpted from *Speaker's Sourcebook II* by Glenn Van Ekeren. ©1993 Glenn Van Ekeren.

Not Without a Fight. Reprinted by permission of Mary Helen Brindell. ©1995 Mary Helen Brindell.

Nintendo Master and *My Hero.* Reprinted by permission of Katie Gill. ©1995 Katie Gill.

Fighting Back—One Man's Battle with a Brain Tumor. Reprinted by permission of Reverend Robert Craig. ©1994 Reverend Robert Craig.

Dare to Dream. Reprinted by permission of Manuel Diotte. ©1994 Manuel Diotte.

Fulfilling My Dreams. Reprinted by permission of Marilyn R. Moody. ©1995 Marilyn R. Moody.

Chris—One Special Fifth-Grader! Reprinted by permission of Louise Biggs. ©1995 Louise Biggs.

Keep on Keeping On. Reprinted by permission of Erik Olesen. ©1995 Erik Olesen.

The Container. Reprinted by permission of The Putnam Publishing Group. Excerpted from *Kitchen Table Wisdom* by Rachel Naomi Remen, M.D. ©1996 Rachel Naomi Remen, M.D.

The Best Day Of My Life. Reprinted by permission of Gregory M. Lousig-Nont. ©1995 Gregory M. Lousig-Nont.

Love Is Stronger . . . and *To the Nurses of the World.* Reprinted by permission of John Wayne Schlatter. ©1995 John Wayne Schlatter.

The Power to Choose. Reprinted by permission of Angela Trafford. ©1995 Sharon Bruckman.

Share the Magic of Chicken Soup

Chicken Soup for the Soul™
101 Stories to Open the Heart and Rekindle the Spirit

The #1 *New York Times* bestseller and ABBY award-winning inspirational book that has touched the lives of millions. Whether you buy it for yourself or as a gift to others, you're sure to enrich the lives of everyone around you with this affordable treasure.

Code 262X: Paperback $12.95
Code 2913: Hardcover $24.00
Code 3812: Large print $16.95

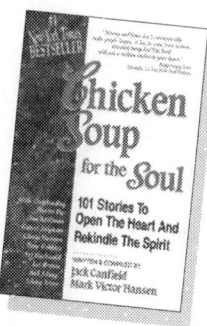

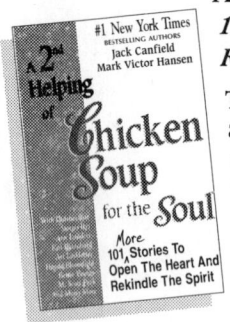

A 2nd Helping of Chicken Soup for the Soul™
101 More Stories to Open the Heart and Rekindle the Spirit

This rare sequel accomplishes the impossible—it is as tasty as the original, and still fat-free. If you enjoyed the first *Chicken Soup for the Soul,* be warned: it was merely the first course in an uplifting grand buffet. These stories will leave you satisfied and full of self-esteem, love and compassion.

Code 3316: Paperback $12.95
Code 3324: Hardcover $24.00
Code 3820: Large print $16.95

A 3rd Serving of Chicken Soup for the Soul™
101 More Stories to Open the Heart and Rekindle the Spirit

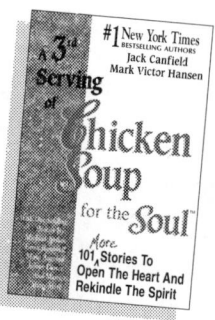

The latest addition to the *Chicken Soup for the Soul* series is guaranteed to put a smile in your heart. Learn through others the important lessons of love, parenting, forgiveness, hope and perseverance. This tasty literary stew will stay with you long after you've put the book down.

Code 3790: Paperback. $12.95
Code 3804: Hardcover. $24.00
Code 4002: Large print $16.95

Available at your favorite bookstore or call
1-800-441-5569 for Visa or MasterCard orders. Prices do not include shipping and handling. Your response code is CSUR.